Gestalt Empty Chair Work

LIBERATING OUR HURT INNER CHILD
TOWARD COMPLETENESS

Additional copies may be ordered from the publisher for educational, business, promotional or premium use.
For information, contact ALIVE Book Publishing at:
alivebookpublishing.com

Book design by Alex P. Johnson

ISBN 13
978-1-63132-238-9
Library of Congress Control Number: 2024916997

Library of Congress Cataloging-in-Publication Data
is available upon request.

First Edition

Published in the United States of America by ALIVE Book Publishing
an imprint of Advanced Publishing LLC
3200 A Danville Blvd., Suite 204, Alamo, California 94507
alivebookpublishing.com

PRINTED IN THE UNITED STATES OF AMERICA

10 9 8 7 6 5 4 3 2 1

Gestalt Empty Chair Work

LIBERATING OUR HURT INNER CHILD
TOWARD COMPLETENESS

*A First-Generation Latino's Journey
of Personal and Professional Growth*

Mario Rivas, Ph.D.
Illustrated by Victoria Bruno

ABOOKS

Alive Book Publishing

Table of Contents

Para mi mama y hermano
que me protegieron y
para mis hijos que me acompanaron

Preface

Self & Others: Why and for Whom
Have I written this Book

"Yo soy Joaquín, perdido en un mundo de confusión: I am Joaquín, lost in a world of confusion . . . "* So goes a famous poem by the Chicano poet Rodolfo Corky Gonzales. The poem tells the experience of how many persons of Mexican descent in the United States often do not experience themselves as part of the social and psychological fabric of our nation. While not of Mexican descent, I am of Latino decent, my parents both being immigrants to the U.S. from Costa Rica, Central America. Nevertheless, here in the U.S.A., I was socialized in great part as Mexican American or Chicano, and I have developed and internalized some of the characteristics of some Mexican Americans, one being not experiencing myself as identifying completely with this nation.

But what I would call my *Mejicano* personal and social psychology is only one self-perception that I hold. I have other self-images that I use to define myself. Specifically, I see part of me as Black or African American. This is because I was raised in North Oakland, California, with many African American friends, families, and mentors. Another part of my self-perception, though, is a mixture of Italian, Irish, Filipino, Asian, Central American and more. My life experience attests to my diverse beginnings in this nation, and how I have travelled on the road to defining my psychological identity as a unique person, including my unique understanding of my world.

Returning to Corky Gonzales, I can truly attest to an early sense of confusion in defining who I am. Importantly, my confusion extended beyond my social realities to my experience within my family, and especially with an abusive father, with having been raised by a single "mama" on welfare, with my lack of a single and secure cultural identify, and with my individual adaptation of my unique psychological challenges in life. That is what this book is about.

Friedrich Hegel, a famous German philosopher, is quoted as saying, "The spirit is never at rest but always engaged in ever progressive motion, in giving itself a new form." Robert Kegan, in his book "The Evolving Self," notes that each one of us is a meaning-maker, and that what we do with meaning is to organize it. He goes on to espouse that psychologically we make meaning, organize, or author a unique self. This self is forever changing. That is what this book is about.

This book is about my organization of self and more pointedly, about my psychological definition of self. My diverse family and social experiences have led me to be who I am, both personally and professionally. My mama is at the core of my caring nature; my diverse social experiences are at the core of my compassionate nature. Together, these two have been central to my "self-authorship" à la Robert Kegan.

But my definition of self has not been a smooth and clear path. I have struggled much with having a place to stand, similar to Jimmy Santiago Baca's psychological journey in his book "A Place to Stand." I have struggled with opening up to my true self because of the confusion I experienced in my early journey to self-identity. That is what this book is about. This book is about how I have opened the emotional gates to defining myself, because e-motions, the "body in motion," are what influence and motivate our journey to self, both with self and with others. And for me, opening the gates to my self-understanding and self-definition have happened in great part because of my experience with Gestalt psychology. That truly is what this book is about! Gestalt psychology is a way of gaining self-knowledge and self-directive action that focuses on identifying, immersing ourselves in, and staying with our emotional selves until we see the clear light of self-understanding, definition, self-direction, and self-action. So in this book I share my personal journey to self-definition from a Gestalt perspective, and I also share my professional journey to compassionately teach and share Gestalt psychology with diverse peoples and communities so that they may have the liberty to define and be the unique individuals they choose to be.

From a teaching perspective, I want to support the personal and professional development of Latin@s and diverse socio-cultural persons through the use of Gestalt psychology, which truly has provided me greater personal freedom to navigate the psychological challenges of my life. I have written what I hope is an intimate and learned book wherein I, a first-generation U.S. Latino, offer firsthand accounts of my efforts to develop my own psychological strength and potential as a person and professional — *mi voz.*

My personal growth in this society has been colored by the Latino lens passed on to me by my mama and the fact that my first language is Spanish. The result of my Latino lens is a perspective of self that has throughout my life always been "different," in that I have not seen the origin of my "self" as completely from U.S. society. Paradoxically, I am a product of the U.S., but more than just a stamp of what generally is seen as the face of our nation, that is, Anglo-American.

I am a true *Estadounidense,* but a citizen of the United States of America with a strong legacy of *Latinismo, Chicanismo,* and multiculturalism, which are identities I gained from the teachings of my mama, as well as personality characteristics I have developed during my social life in the U.S. My intention is to share what I have discovered about how to develop one's potential as a person, which sadly I have done primarily through the use of trial and error. I want to help you, the reader, to lessen the amount of trial and error in your life so that you may benefit from my search for happiness, personal peace, and success as a person and professional.

In hundreds of presentations about personal development that I have given in high schools, community colleges, universities, community agencies, community groups, and conferences, I begin by citing the following anonymous quote: "Everybody is born unique!" Surprisingly, audiences unanimously agree with this quote. However, the majority of persons also agree with exasperation when they hear the second half of the quote: "But, most of us die copies!" All born unique, but most die copies. Hmmm, what's going on here?

Discussion of this quote leads to the conclusion that people give up living out their uniqueness because of one main factor — fear (in Spanish, *miedo*): fear to be different; fear of not being accepted by others; fear of rejection; fear of not trusting to experiment to learn what is correct for the self. This book, then, is about the challenge for each of us to be who we are rather than who we should be or need to be, that is, to be our true, hopefully complete, selves. Questions that have challenged me in my life, and ones that I hope to clarify follow: What is our true self? Our unique self? Our complete self?

In talks I also share the following well-known quote of Dr. Fritz Perls, the creator of Gestalt therapy: "It is our

birthright to achieve completeness!" Yes! is the refrain from
all audiences. But what does it mean to achieve completeness? And does achieving completeness mean being our
unique self? I will write to integrate the latter quotes to paint
a picture of how thinking, feeling, and acting our unique
selves is possibly the main aspect of our achieving completeness. In this regard, from the outset, I share that I see becoming complete as a person as a "way of being," rather than a
specific goal or accomplishment.

Nevertheless, I believe that "being complete" does have
component parts; however, the essence of being complete is
about doing, doing, doing — doing oneself! I am reminded
of a quote attributed to the Greek philosopher Socrates: "To
be is to do." Here is the core of what I want to share about
being our unique self and achieving completeness as a person: We must act consistent with how we uniquely experience ourselves and the world around us if we are to live
fully, and thereby move to becoming psychologically complete as a human being.

As I emphasize action as the core of being a complete
person, I want to share how I have come to know, feel, act,
and do myself more and more over time. In this regard, the
following is a Spanish phrase that I have developed to describe what to be or act oneself means: "*Saber, Entender, Sentir, Escoger, y Hacer*" — "Know, Understand, *Feel*, Choose,
and Act." I have come to understand this phrase both from
the study of psychology and the experience of Gestalt personal development therapy, as well as constantly reflecting
on my daily actions. The emphasis on the italicized word
"feel" is important because at the center to be oneself is to
feel or experience the unique emotions of our oneness — of
our unified body and mind.

I begin this book in my seventy-first year, and I write both as one who has attained a substantial level of knowledge about what is meant by being alive, and at the same time, as one who continually seeks the meaning of my life. I continue to search and strive to be my uniqueness and completeness. As such, in my many hours of Gestalt personal development work, I have formed and continue to form clarity and personal meaning of confusing emotions and related thoughts and images that have come to signify the story of my life, what many philosophers and psychologists call the theme or script of one's life.

This book tells how I have lived life, learning gradually to express my "self" (think, feel and behave) as honestly as possible, as a person and through my profession as teacher and psychologist, sharing what I have learned so others can be more capable to live their vision of a fulfilling life. My focus is twofold: (1) Communicate knowledge to individuals and groups that often do not experience the benefits of studying psychology and personal development methods; and (2) Inspire Latin@s (a combined form of Latino and Latina), other persons of color, professionals, and volunteers providing psychological education to underserved diverse communities to use Gestalt personal development methods to facilitate personal growth in individuals and groups.

I seek to reach persons who have never heard about fascinating centers of personal development such as the Esalen Institute in Big Sur, California, or Spirit Rock in Woodacre, California, or who have never read the ideas of such renowned Gestalt therapists as Fritz Perls, Joseph Zinker, Bud Feder, Erving and Marie Polster, Muriel Schiffman, Anne Teachworth, and many others. At the same time, I want to acknowledge the wisdom of Dr. Abe Levitsky, a loving

Gestalt therapist with whom I did personal development work in Berkeley, California, who admonished, "Mario, it's not all about Gestalt." Certainly, Abe. I agree, (and I miss you very much); however, for me, Gestalt work has been the central force for my personal psychological development.

As it has been for me, the power of psychology to help people live fulfilling lives reaches beyond Gestalt therapy to such wise persons as Erik Erikson ("Childhood and Society"), Rick Hanson and Richard Mendius ("Buddha's Brain"), Ken Keyes ("Handbook to Higher Consciousness), Carl Rogers ("On Becoming a Person," "Person to Person" "Freedom to Learn"), Karen Horney ("Our Inner Conflicts"), William Schutz ("Joy," "Here Comes Everybody," "The Human Element"), Sheldon Kopp ("If You Meet the Buddha on the Road, Kill Him!"), Robert Kegan ("The Evolving Self," "Immunity to Change"), Nathaniel Branden (The Six Pillars of Self Esteem," "The Psychology of Self-Esteem"), Eric Berne ("Transactional Analysis"; "Games People Play"), and Thomas Harris ("I'm OK—You're OK"), and more.

Nevertheless, in this book I want to share how Gestalt methods have helped me, a first-generation Latino in the U.S., to learn to experience and know my "self," and to help seekers of personal development to become knowledgeable of Gestalt personal growth methods that influenced my potential and capacity for personal fulfillment and professional development.

My teaching is for all persons who have asked me what books to read to become more knowledgeable about psychology and personal development (many that I have named in the preceding paragraph). Related to approaching

this book, what comes to mind for me is what Mortimer
Adler wrote in his book "How to Read a Book." He wrote
that after reading a book we should be able to distill the essential content down to one sentence. Therefore, I want to
attempt at the beginning to write one sentence that tells
what this book is about. Here goes:

Our adult confidence and ability to support our unique
self to face life's challenges is too often damaged by fears
learned in childhood, doubts and shame about how to handle
difficult life situations; the negative emotions from childhood are internalized in unconscious body-mind memories
and related images, and Gestalt personal development
methods can be used to address through awareness these
internalized fears and revitalize the adults' body-mind ability to act responsibly and effectively to complete oneself as
a unique human being!

From the beginning, it is also my intention to write this
book in Spanish, my first language, because I want Spanish-
speaking people all over the U.S., Latin America, and the
world to have access to the knowledge I have gained by
studying psychology, and in particular, Gestalt personal development concepts and methods of personal growth. I have
spent a good deal of my professional life working with
Latin@s in and out of the U.S., and I have found that the
ideas and methods that I will share in this book are very useful to Latin@s (now sometimes labeled Latinx) groups and
individuals, such as volunteer counselors at Bay Area
Women Against Rape (BAWAR), Ms. Yuselin Martinez'
community personal growth groups, which she offers in
and around Oakland, California, Randy Menjivar's Latino
groups at Unity High School in East Oakland, California,
and the teens and adults of CRECE (Central American

Refugee Committee), a Nicaraguan community organization, also in East Oakland, California.

At its core, this book also reflects a value taught to me by my Costa Rican mama, Josefina Mata Trejos Rivas: "*Lo mas importante en la vida es ayudar a nuestro projimo*" — the most important thing in life is to help our fellow human beings. *Si, si, si, mamasita!* This book is about giving back to others what I have been so fortunate to learn about psychology and personal growth, especially because I come from a background that generally does not expose persons like me to the tremendous possibilities that exist in our world for psychological growth.

My mother, a Costa Rican Latina with a six-grade education who raised my brother, Francisco, and me, while working as a maid and house cleaner in Oakland, California, wanted me to be a Lasallian Christian Brother and teacher (with concern for the poor, and social justice). She wanted me to be like Saint John Bosco, to be concerned for the learning needs of children. In great part, I have lived out my mother's dreams, but not as a Christian Brother or priest; rather, I have become a teacher of psychology who helps others learn how to develop their human potential to live more complete and satisfying lives.

This book for me also reflects one of the most powerful avenues for psychological learning and growth: honest personal sharing. In this regard, I will share psychological challenges that I've encountered related to my maturing and becoming complete, as a Latino and as a unique person living in the U.S., as well as describing how I have used Gestalt personal development psychology to support my journey and the journey of others to personal and professional growth. I focus on the psychology of being human. This psychology is one wherein I see the meaning of being a human is to be (not have) an effective "self" who thinks, feels, and acts according to personally relevant and life-clarifying values and beliefs, and according to ways of being that lead in the direction of living in a physically and psychologically (unified body-mind) effective and complete way. Importantly, in this book I make few arguments about how a person should be; rather, I offer a "way" for people to move forward to have balance within themselves, including clarity of thinking, expressiveness of one's body, and self-directedness, qualities which I feel are necessary for choosing a life that is true and supportive of how one wants to be. I leave it to each of you to choose your unique road in life.

Personally, I share that my psychological challenges related to developing the unique person I am stem from coming from an abusive family situation in my early years, with a family-punishing father, and extending to being raised on welfare from age nine in North Oakland, California by a loving, mono-lingual Spanish-speaking mother who raised my slightly older brother (eleven months), Franklin/Frank/Francisco, and myself, while working every day as a maid and house cleaner. My family-punishing father gave me a legacy of fear and doubt that I would have to learn how to face, understand, and integrate into a resilient and stronger self. My fearful, loving mother, who was experiencing daily the constant anxiety as a single Latina "mama," especially one who is not loved and supported by her husband, often faces in raising children — alone in a country not her own she gave me a legacy of mixed fear, hope, personal strength, and love that would eventually support me to learn how to construct a solid Latino foundation to build a self who could think, speak up, and work to own his true feelings, thoughts, and actions.

My professional and volunteer work with others, Latin@s, Chican@s, African Americans, Filipinos, Asians, and European-Americans, of all ages and genders, is also chronicled in this book through my sharing about how I learned to develop the competence to help others understand and choose paths of growth in life by using the resources of psychology, and especially Gestalt therapy theory and practice related to personal development. With respect to helping others grow, I share personal development work that I have done with others wherein they "unbind" themselves from their too often negative family, childhood, and societal self-limiting legacies, which restrict personal insight and effective action to live life as self-understanding and self-directing persons.

I want to highlight that my personal growth and efforts to support the development of others has been affected by having grown up as a first-generation Latino in the U.S. Our society is in development much like all of us, with tugs and pulls that come from many forces: clashing diverse cultures, different religious perspectives, economic inequalities, political divisiveness, racial strife, racist attitudes, and many other challenges which generally are factors that do not offer a clear path or fertile ground for finding and being oneself. Rather, our divergent society too often puts roadblocks in front of individual efforts, especially for persons of color, to truly direct ourselves in ways that support developing our "real self."

Finally, a note about why the focus on Gestalt personal development concepts is the central theme in the organization of this book. For one, Gestalt personal development concepts have proven to be the most powerful ideas and related personal growth methods that have made a difference in my psychological development, as well as the work I have done in supporting the psychological growth of thousands of persons I have had the good fortune to help in and around the San Francisco-Oakland Bay Area, and across the United States. In my own development, Gestalt personal development work has provided me with a conceptual and experiential understanding for how to grow to be satisfied with how I want to and how I actually live my life. Similarly, in my support of others' personal growth, Gestalt methods have proven the most useful in impacting the growth of others. With respect to helping the psychological growth of others, I share that I have often been told by many persons that my one Gestalt Educational Counseling (GEC) intervention, which I will share in this book, has been more beneficial than months and even years of therapy!

So, my intent in this book is to share what I have learned firsthand about personal growth, as well as what I have learned about how to help others grow and find life satisfaction, especially again, from a Gestalt perspective. Along with sharing what I have learned, I will share the "how" of Gestalt personal development methods, including specifics about how Gestalt personal development methods work. I will also share how I have used Gestalt personal development methods in my work with community college and university students, and in my volunteer work with Latin@ community groups in and around Oakland, California.

Chapter 1

**Gestalt Psychology Opens a Gate to My Emotions and
Sparks a Clarity of Growth in My Life**

It was 1992, and I was forty-five years old. I had progressed
to the position of Associate Dean of Undergraduate Studies
at San Francisco State University, but still, I was nervous a
lot in my work and life, not unlike how I had been as a little
boy, a teenager, and a young adult. I had completed a doctorate at the University of Minnesota, but I was not at peace.
I had a lovely family, including a wife and four children, but
I knew that some part of me was not complete. I wanted to
grow, develop my ability to be personally and professionally satisfied, and completely happy. I did not want to continue a life of internal personal struggle with what outside
seemed like a satisfied and successful person.

I remember when I gave talks to high school students
throughout San Francisco, I would say, "This little first-generation Latino welfare kid whose mother was a maid has
risen to be a dean at San Francisco State University, and you
too can achieve good things for yourself!" Also, I recall with
fondness, a ninth grade African American youngster from
San Francisco's McAteer High School who came up to me
after a presentation and told me that he had enjoyed my
talk.

I asked, "What did you like?"

He answered, using and placing his hands near the
ground, standing on his tip toes and raising his other hand
to the sky to emphasize his words, "Because you went from
nothing to something!"

But still, inside, I did not completely feel my "something." I had not truly achieved an inner "something" to give me peace. Part of me was shaky and nervous, and incomplete. I was searching for something more within me!

I decided there and then to face myself, to learn definitively how to understand my emotions and grow as a person and achieve peace, happiness, and satisfaction. But, how? But, how? I breathe deeply in the present moment as I remember myself at that time; I breathe deeply because I see the goodness of that moment when I listened to my inner need for personal growth.

I recall that I revisited all my past efforts to develop my psychological potential, and what stood out was a time at the University of Minnesota when I similarly was searching for what I considered my "stronger, clearer, and more complete" self. Then I decided to take a course in Gestalt personal development with Dr. Bart Grossman, a well-known Gestalt therapist. It was then that I opened the gate to my true emotional self, as well as catching a glimpse of my path toward personal growth. However, in that class my path of bettering myself was not a straight and complete one, because even though I had a powerful growth experience, I did not continue to pursue Gestalt personal development work outside the class. I did not follow through. But five years later, I was now ready to step into Gestalt in a complete way, so I searched the internet and saw an advertisement for the Gestalt Institute of San Francisco. I made a call, and there I truly began my Gestalt personal and professional journey to my completeness as a person, of which this book is about.

I want to start with a small preview regarding how Gestalt personal development methods work, especially regarding the importance of the connection between feeling, thinking, and behaving. The Gestalt approach to personal development involves "staying with" one's experience of self in order to develop greater awareness about where we get stuck in thinking, feeling, and acting our unique self. "Staying with self" involves remaining in a particular difficult emotional space, rather than moving over one's experiences without truly feeling the impact of a particular emotional experience. "Staying with oneself" means paying attention to what one is thinking, feeling, and doing in any given moment. This is not an easy process, because often we learn in our life to defend our psychological self by avoiding or blocking our ability to be aware of what we are actually experiencing in a given situation.

In this regard, when doing Gestalt work and "getting stuck" in not being able to have a clear awareness of one's experience, the person guiding you may ask you what visual image comes to your mind associated with your emotional state. This is a powerful experience, because visual images associated with emotional states often connect one to early life experiences that help us become more aware of certain themes in our life or our "life script," that may be affecting our present functioning. However, getting unstuck when one is emotionally overwhelmed is not always an easy proposition.

As such, when I have been "stuck" while doing Gestalt work, I often have asked myself, "What is the meaning of the images that emerge from the background of my life?" By way of example, one of the major and initially confusing images that emerged for me when being stuck in a difficult emotional state was an image involving an undefined mixture of turbulent, disordered, unformed, and a meaningless jumble of chaotic pictures similar to the image of many cartoon fights that I watched on television in my childhood.

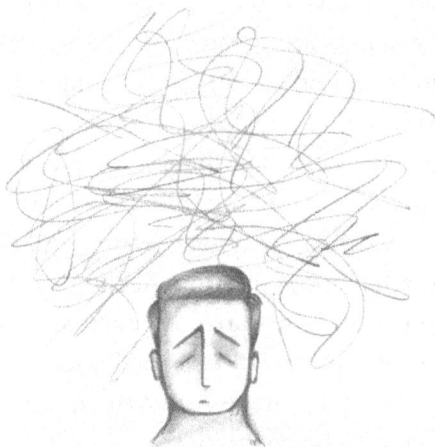

This figure kept coming up over and over in my imagination when during my personal development work I was asked to identify a picture or image from my life that connected to my present emotional upheaval. This was a very significant experience for me as I searched for the strength to face and understand challenging emotions and personal reactions to my life such as fear, doubt, unsteadiness, indecision, and anger. Literally, in my imagination, this was the picture I saw over and over again when asked to connect my experience of difficult feelings with a particular visual image: "What image do you see and connect to your present emotions?"

As I "stayed with this cartoon-like image," and felt it more and more, the next figure that came into my awareness when asked to "stay with the emotions that went with the chaotic jumble cartoon-like picture," was that of frighteningly sharp teeth. Truly, I experienced a very raw fear when this image came to my mind.

Eventually, I came to see that these teeth were part of the scary growl of a fierce and angry dog. This dog, I imagined,

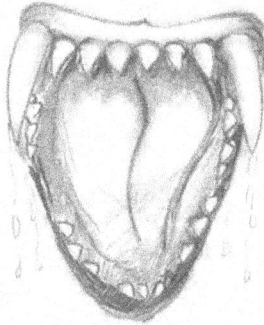

was fearful to approach or touch. Still, I experimented with my imagination and related feelings, and more and more I contacted the fear connected with imagining to reach out to touch the dog's head. One day, I reached out in my imagination, and slightly touched a tough, rock-hard head. Ugh! Yuk! It was so hard! In time, what came next was the image of a strong, firm, assured, and calm dog stolidly sitting on his hind legs, guarding something or someone behind him.

With more "work," I began to see that in the "background" of this figure was my "little Mario" self with a

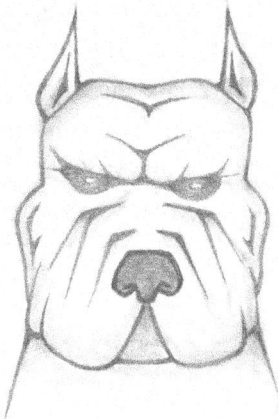

tummy protruding from his green-and-yellow-striped T shirt, standing in front of a little wood structure in El Tejar, Costa Rica, a small town where I lived part of my childhood. The little boy was alone, yet not alone; tentative, but not lost. Also, not complete!

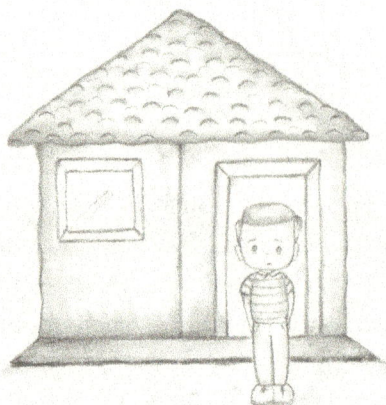

From the image of this little boy, what I have come to call my "Childhood Legacy," has come, through many hours of Gestalt personal development work, an alternating figure of the small child and a fully formed man, parent, and professional — a person becoming complete. That is what this book is about: Learning to use the Gestalt psychological approach to clarify the unique person I am and who you are by becoming aware of how our personalities are primarily formed from our childhood experiences and how through awareness we can know and become who we are and want to be.

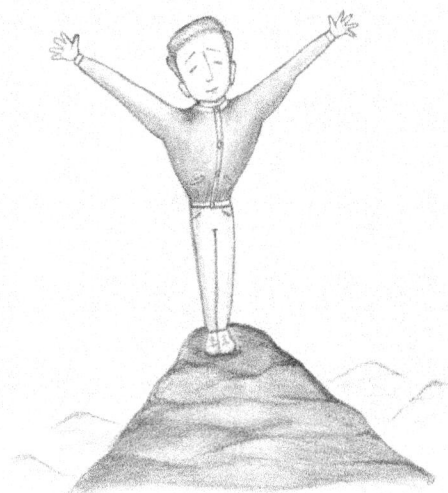

Chapter 2

Fourteen Gestalt Ideas for Understanding One's Emotions and Development as a Person

- *The Meaning of Gestalt*
- *The First and Foremost Gestalt: I am "Some<u>body</u>"*
- *Gestalt Cycle of Experience — Awareness and Integration of Our Unique Experience of Self: Sensation, Awareness, Mobilization of Energy, Contact, Assimilation, Withdrawal*
- *The Gestalt of Self-Support: From Other Support to Self-Support*
- *The Gestalt "Shame Bind:" Backing Away, and Not Leaning Forward into Life*
- *Body Armor*
- *Mind-Body Associational Images*
- *The "Empty Chair" Technique: Integrating Weakness and Strength/Building Self-Support*
- *Doing Gestalt Experiments to Test Out Gestalts*
- *Building Awareness of One's Process of Forming Gestalts*
- *The Concepts of Figure and Ground and Becoming Aware of Gestalt Formation*
- *"Staying" with" Difficult Sensations Until We are Able to Develop Gestalts of Self-support*
- *The Gestalt of Completing I: Experiencing CONTACT with My Growing, Learning Self*
- *Unfinished Gestalts are "Unfinished Business" and the Development of Our Unique Self*

I want to give a brief introduction to Gestalt personal development concepts to orient you to ideas that I will explain in this book related to my personal and professional growth, as well as how I support others to develop psychologically through Gestalt personal development methods (called "work"). I will use some of the Gestalt concepts as chapter headings to point the way to how Gestalt methods relate to my (our) personal and professional growth. I will continue referring to Gestalt principles throughout the book: (1) To help you have a greater understanding for how Gestalt personal development ideas and methods can help each of us grow psychologically; and (2) How I apply these ideas and methods in supporting the personal and professional growth of students and persons in various communities. Importantly, my description of the following concepts reflects how I understand these principles. For more clarity, you can do further reading in many books that cover Gestalt therapy.

The Meaning of Gestalt

The Merriam-Webster definition of the word Gestalt is: "An organized whole that is perceived to be more than the sum of its parts." As a psychological personal development concept, a Gestalt is an individual experience wherein a person interacts with any life situation and forms a unique understanding or reaction (thoughts, feelings, and behaviors) that changes the experience, meaning, and organization of a person's sense of self. For me, the idea of Gestalt also relates to the forming of a sense of self that is more complete or whole. The experience of Gestalt formation can either be positive or negative. When positive, a Gestalt is completed or experienced as a whole, and leads to expanded development and clarity regarding the organization and experience of the self. When negative, a Gestalt is not completed, and leads to an "unfinished situation" ("unfinished business" in Gestalt parlance) wherein the individual's sense of self does not become clearer, and psychological growth is not experienced fully.

In the process of experiencing Gestalt formation and completing Gestalts, we can learn either to have greater "self-support" to assist us to develop our unique sense of self, or we can form incomplete Gestalts that can undermine or get in the way of developing our uniqueness. In short, from birth we are constantly forming Gestalts to make sense of our self in the world. This is an ongoing process that continues throughout life, because life is a never-ending journey of learning and continual personal growth. However, personal growth is not guaranteed; sometimes our growth is frustrated, and often growth demands effort and hard work, which is very, very challenging emotionally, behaviorally, and cognitively.

The following is a thematic example of the formation of an incomplete Gestalt in a person's childhood experience that I have witnessed countless times when counseling individuals, which I have seen to be harmful to the development of a strong or confident sense of self: A child experiences his parents in a loud argument regarding their relationship, wherein the child has no power to make the situation better. The incomplete Gestalt that I have seen formed by the child (which is too often carried as part of the personality into adulthood) involves the child perceiving and experiencing his or her "self" as incapable of having a sense of safety and confidence in the environment, and unable to handle the fear and confusion of the family situation.

This very often leads to the child perceiving his or her "self" as unlovable and not supported in his or her growth as a person.

In his book "I'm OK; Your OK," Dr. Thomas Harris would label this child's perspective as "I'm not OK!" Importantly, the incomplete Gestalt that is formed in this situation affects the child's self-concept, their perception of self and self-esteem- how the child feels about their self-concept. Finally, and very important related to the formation of the self-Gestalt, the child embodies in his/her central nervous system (brain and spinal cord) and body (nerves, muscles, and glands), a concentration of negative physical and chemical energy that gets in the way of the individual acting in self-supporting and self-enhancing ways (see "The Body Keeps the Score" by Bessel Van Der Kolk, M.D. for an excellent explanation of this phenomena). An incomplete Gestalt is distinguished from a complete Gestalt in that the latter resolves a life challenge in a way that results in the individual being more complete as a person and more capable of effectively supporting the self to live life in a satisfying and growth-oriented manner.

The First and Foremost Gestalt: I am "Somebody"

We are "somebody" means just that: who we are is internalized, embodied in the wholeness of our physical self (Kurt Goldstein's concept of the "organism as a whole"). For me, the concept of "wholeness" is of huge importance because it reflects our biological move towards integration of self, which begins at conception, and continues in the womb and into our on-going development as human beings. The Gestalt phrase, "It is our birthright to achieve completeness," is a direct expression of our human need to integrate our self or to move toward completeness. In the womb, the fetus has reflexes (e.g., the Moro reflex), and after birth our reflexes (e.g., the rooting reflex, startle reflex, etc.) are our inherited way of adapting and learning to be effective in the world. Underlying this motion toward integration is the biology of our brain progressively becoming more complete through the accumulation of more and more neurons (cells that specialize in communication and organizing information) in our brain (eventually, all of us have one-hundred billion neurons!). Importantly, as we add more and more neurons, we biologically become more integrated (whole) as an organism that can adapt more effectively to our environment.

Psychologically, the term "Gestalt" refers to an underlying motion in our psychology that moves us to completing situations in our daily lives, and to completing ourselves as psychologically aware human beings. The completeness or incompleteness of Gestalts are very important to our psychological health because the more we can gain completeness in daily life situations, the more we become more whole as a person. Our mind-body relationship is key to forming Gestalts. Our mind forms understandings of our experiences, and our stored "body emotions" or habitual somatic reactions, are expressions of complete or incomplete gestalts that we have each formed in our lives. When we respond to life situations, our reactions are our self-Gestalt (mind-body reactions) as to how we experience and interpret the world. Our self-Gestalt can be one where we "lean into life," as Dr. Abe Levitsky used to say to me in therapy sessions, with energy, creativity, and support for one's growth, or our self-Gestalt can be one where we stifle, back away, or avoid, that is, not support ourselves to lean positively into the challenges of life, à la Lee and Wheeler's "Voice of Shame."

With respect to our body, Fritz Perls wrote in his book "Gestalt Therapy Verbatim," that we intrinsically have within our minds and bodies, are born with what he calls, "organismic self-regulation," which is the built-in or natural ability, developed over thousands of years of evolution, of our mind and body to cope with and adapt effectively to life. If we trust our organism, our mind-body, we will progressively create effective growth-oriented Gestalts which will support us to use our human wisdom to choose and act according to how we want to actualize our self (be the some-body we want to be). Importantly, trusting our organism in our life involves what Perls calls "self-supportive breathing." Anxiety is "excitement without oxygen;" when we breathe in the midst of difficult challenges, we support ourselves to access our intrinsic life energy to act and experiment with different options for handling and resolving the challenges of life, i.e., complete Gestalts in an effective manner.

Gestalt Cycle of Experience: Awareness and Integration of Our Unique Experience of Self

For me, there are two well-known psychological quotes essential to understanding the core of Gestalt personal growth concepts. One is by Stanley Keleman, who titled his book with it: "Your Body Speaks Its Mind." The other is by Fritz Perls, who wrote, "It is our birthright to achieve completeness." Both of these ideas tie to the meaning of the word Gestalt, that is, a whole or entirety of some thought or action/experience. As humans, we are one living being, one whole, comprised of a potentially unified, integrated mind and body. As humans, the highest level of our being is to be whole and complete, or in general terms, be who we are.

Gertrude Stein wrote, "A rose is a rose is a rose," which in Gestalt parlance is called the law of identity: We are what we are! Perls wrote that an eagle soars, not because it accepts or thinks of itself as an eagle. No, an eagle soars because that is what it is. Humans are analogous to an eagle, that is, we have an essence. According to Gestalt philosophy, the essence of being human is to be who we are. In short, we are here to complete ourselves as we uniquely are and as such, to strive every moment of our lives to achieve completeness of functioning as a human being.

So, what does it mean to be our "self" from a Gestalt perspective? It means to be an integrated whole in thinking, feeling, and behaving. In his book "Creative Process in Gestalt Therapy," Joseph Zinker described what he called the "Gestalt Cycle of Experience," wherein he outlined the process that we go through in our daily existence as we work to be conscious, aware of ourselves, and to complete our unique "self." The cycle describes an individual's movement from sensing the world, to becoming aware of how our sense-making experience (body and mind) reflect our unique desires, needs, and wants, mobilizing our energy to move toward meeting our needs and desires, to actual directed action toward satisfying what it is we need and want. And then, to having contact with our individually unique experiencing of self-in-action and, finally, to arrive to the point of assimilating or integrating each of our ongoing life experiences with a greater sense of who we are.

This is the Gestalt Cycle of Experience: feeling our self and acting our self, all in the process of progressively knowing, defining, and becoming who we uniquely are. Importantly, this process of knowing and becoming our self is organismic, that is, based in the biology of what is the essence of being a human being. In short, we as humans have evolved to make meaningful Gestalts in the world; we have evolved to be an organism that moves toward being integrated and complete as the unique person we each are. This moving toward completing our unique self is also called "self-realization."

What follows is an expansion of each of the steps in the Gestalt Cycle of Experience. I use select Gestalt concepts to explain the meaning and importance of each step in the cycle with respect to our personal development, integration, and realization of a complete self.

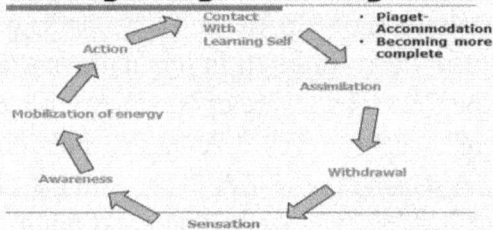

The Gestalt Cycle of Experience: Integrating "Learning Self"

Adapted from "The Creative Process in Gestalt Therapy," by Joseph Zinker, 2006.

Sensation

Our mind and body as one unity is our embodied sense of self. Through evolution, our body-mind developed to "make sense" of the world. First, we use our senses to perceive and respond to what emerges as important in our life, our "emergencies." If there is danger and we sense danger, we respond with some behavior to protect our self; if we sense that something or someone is good for us, we move with energy to receive or partake of the experience. Our senses are our connection to life. In the Gestalt Cycle of Experience, our senses are the first step in the cycle that signals to us that we have a need or want that comes either from within, e.g., the need for food, sleep, sex, etc., or signals that there is a need or want that results from our interaction with our environment, e.g., the need to protect self when there is danger or need to open up to others when there is love, acceptance, etc.

If we are open to our senses, our sense-making experience, we begin every experience with movement toward understanding and meeting the needs and wants of what emerges as important in our life. Sadly, we can learn through negative life experiences, especially in our childhood, to not listen or to not trust or be fearful of our sense-making experience, and when this occurs, we become a person less able to move into and along the Gestalt Cycle of Experience. In these instances, we learn to not open up to and not trust our senses. We therefore are hampered in our ability to initiate actions leading to greater clarity of experiencing self and the environment around us.

Awareness

When we accept and identify what our senses communicate to us, we have awareness. We therefore continue along the cycle and move to taking action to meet our needs and wants. If we have learned not to value, be fearful of, or not trust what our senses communicate to us, we will stop our movement through the Gestalt Cycle of Experience. For example, if in childhood I am abused in some way and I become fearful of standing up for myself, I may shut down my sense-making self when I want to assert and support myself because I am being lessened by the way others are treating me. Or possibly, and even worse, subconsciously, I may shut down my senses when psychologically from within I am being unduly critical or negative toward myself.

An example of this is an instance when my senses are signaling that I need to cry and feel hurt or angry for the manner I am being treated, and instead of accepting and supporting my inchoate tears or acknowledging and supporting the anger in my arms, I may stop myself from feeling anything. Another example may be that I may misinterpret my senses as communicating to me that I should harm myself versus be angry toward others. If I lack awareness or clarity for what my senses are communicating to me, I cannot move through the Gestalt Cycle of Experience to meet my true needs and wants.

Mobilization of Energy

Now, if I have clarity with the experience of my senses as well as awareness of what my senses are communicating to me related to what I need and want, I can mobilize my energy to move toward satisfying ongoing life needs and wants. Were life so simple! Very often we learn, either from our own misinterpretations of life experiences or by imposition of the ideas and will of others for how life should be (should-isms), to not mobilize our energy to act in ways to benefit meeting our needs or to support us to learn to act in ways to effectively meet our needs and wants.

Mobilization of energy is a felt experience. Our body mobilizes physical energy that is aimed at action. Our shoulders, arms, legs, etc. are energized to act. We *feel* ourselves wanting to move in specific ways that aim toward satisfying some physical or psychological need or want. Examples of this are when we tighten our jaw, clench our fists, have shaky legs, or cover our eyes with our hands. In each of these instances, we are communicating a message to our self with our body that we need to take some form of action to meet our needs, wants, and desires. The challenge is to learn to trust what our body is trying to communicate, and experiment with actions in life to learn to understand how our body's reactions are attempts to form positive Gestalts in support of our personal growth.

Action

"To be is to do," wrote William James, often called the father of American psychology. James was not a Gestalt psychologist; however, from a Gestalt perspective, "action" is that part of the Gestalt Cycle of Experience where we test our view or perspective of our self in the world. From sensing to becoming aware of what our senses are communicating to us and responding to our needs and wants, we can behave or act on what our body and mind as one is communicating to us and, therefore, we can move closer to understanding what is important and necessary for us to complete our meaning of who we are and what we want out of life. To act on what we sense as important to meet our individual needs and wants in the world is central to defining and becoming who we uniquely are. Action is life: when we act, we can learn from the outcomes of our actions what is important to us and what makes us feel more complete as a unique individual.

Contact

When we act on what our sense-making-self signals as something necessary to satisfy our experienced needs, we move along the Gestalt Cycle of Experience to have knowledge of what is unique to us about what are our needs and wants — what we value and who we are. Each action we take can move us closer and closer to defining who we are and what is uniquely different or special about our self. In the latter sentence, the meaning of the word "can," is essential, because defining our uniqueness is not a cause-and-effect phenomenon where all action leads to greater clarity as to who we are and what is unique about our needs and wants. Our actions can lead to greater clarity about our unique self, but that depends on whether or not we have been given environmental support throughout our life, especially in childhood, to learn to trust and use our sense-making ability to act and be who we want to be.

If we have learned to trust and support our definition of what is important in life to us, each action is more than likely freely chosen to move toward meeting our needs and wants. Contact, in this sense, is when as individuals we experience contact with experience inside and outside of ourselves that adds clarity and completeness to what is unique about us. Importantly, contact is also a felt experience; our mind-body experiences our self-in-action. We grow - we move to be complete!

Assimilation

Assimilation is that part of the Gestalt Cycle of Experience where we assimilate or integrate new information or knowledge about our unique experience of self, and experience our mind and body as one. Assimilation is that part of the cycle where we integrate or unite our experience into the meaning and "oneness" of who we are. We feel, think, and act as one; we are an integrated whole. In his book "In and Out the Garbage Pail," Fritz Perls distinguishes between our "true selves" versus the self who lives to meet the demands of others. If again, our environment, especially in our formative years, has supported us to trust and act on our sense-making ability to know and act on what are truly our needs and wants, who we really are, we will act in ways that move us closer and closer to clarity about what is our "center" as a person. The more clarity we have about what is the core of our true self, the more we will act in ways to support who it is we are, à la "a rose is a rose is a rose" — we are who we are! Again, sadly, if we do not trust our sense-making ability, we will often fearfully move away from supporting the knowing and development of our "true self." Instead, we will become alienated from what is the essence of who we are; we will not support ourselves to move through or complete our Gestalt Cycle of Experience.

Withdrawal

Our experience of life is an endless series of emerging experiences or as is known in Gestalt terms, emergencies. A new experience initiates a new Gestalt Cycle of Experience, each one leading to either the possibility of less or more clarity regarding who we are. Each experience is a Gestalt or a whole, wherein the experience can be completed and help us move toward greater clarity and completeness of our true self, or not be completed, and therefore, frustrate our movement toward completing our self, à la, "It is our birthright to achieve completeness." Experiences where we do not support our self to move through the cycle are known as "incomplete Gestalts" or "unfinished business." Incomplete Gestalts create holes in the development of our completeness as a person. Every emergency offers the possibility of getting to know and act as our true selves. So it is that whether we complete or not complete each of our life emergencies, we nevertheless move on in life to live with more clarity and completeness, or less clarity and completeness. The experience of completeness or incompleteness are also felt experiences!

The Gestalt of Self-Support: Developing From Other Support to Self-Support

"Self-support" is a Gestalt concept meaning that we develop or internalize, make part of ourselves, the ability to assume direct responsibility for facing and taking on our life challenges. Self-support does not mean that we do everything alone; rather, when we face challenges, we rely on ourselves to act and move in the direction that we need to in order to develop our unique potential. We may turn to others either because we know we need other's support to move forward in our lives, or we may choose to act independently to address our life challenges. Self-support means that we do not turn away from ourselves because we experience a feeling or perception of lack of potential to act productively and competently. Instead, self-support means that we accept and experience ourselves as we are, and we move forward, even indirectly or haltingly, trusting that we can act to resolve our personal development challenges, our "emergencies."

Self-support is a personal attribute that in childhood we need support from significant others, parents, guides, family members to develop. If support from others does not occur in our early life, we can develop a Gestalt where we experience self with doubt, shame, lack of ability, and more. This negative self-Gestalt is often carried into adulthood as a "shame bind," where we may back away from supporting our self to assume personal responsibility to face the challenges of life. Shame binds are felt experiences when we do not accept or trust the inborn ability to "lean into" challenges that emerge in our life.

The Gestalt "Shame Bind:" Backing Away, and Not Leaning Forward into Life

In "The Voice of Shame," edited by Robert Lee and Gordon Wheeler, Lee describes a process whereby we develop what in Gestalt terms is called "shame binds." Shame binds are just that, feelings of shame that bind us with feelings of hopelessness, doubt, and worthlessness. These shame binds lessen our ability to rely on self-support and, instead, lead us to turn away from the world rather than lean forward into life when we have difficult psychological challenges and emergencies.

Where do these shame binds originate? How do they develop? Shame binds in great part form in childhood, but can originate whenever we are psychologically vulnerable. In the case of shame binds, a challenging situation comes up when we need love, support, understanding, or encouragement from self or others. For example, in one situation we may be abused, and therefore develop a shame bind where we experience the world as a hostile, dangerous place where we are incapable of experiencing safety and hope for a good life. Or, in another situation, as when parents are constantly fighting or going through separation or divorce, we as a child may think and feel that the world is a hopeless place where we have no ability to correct what is occurring in our life.

In such situations, we have a need to feel strong, as if we can produce a positive effect on the world, or we may want others to provide a sense of strength, security, and safety for us. In such difficult life situations, we want to reach out to others in hope of experiencing a positive interaction where we are valued, loved, respected, understood, supported to understand the challenges we are facing, and helped to feel that the situation is not totally hopeless — e.g., losing our family or losing connection with a parent does not necessarily mean a total loss of the love, understanding, and support which are necessary to grow and develop strength as a person. Instead of a positive experience, too often we experience non-supportive, negative responses from our surrounding environment, and experience ourselves as not being able to effectively reach out to the world for the sense of support that we need. The result is that we withdraw from such experiences with a feeling of hopelessness, incompetence, lack of feeling valued, or lack of self-respect, e.g., we can feel shame about who we are. This experience becomes part of our body.

Shame binds are not all-powerful; they can be overcome, and for me, the best way has been to do Gestalt "Empty

Chair" work, where the person with a shame bind re-experiences, the early situation using the support of their adult self and the care and support of a counselor, therapist, or from supportive group participants who provides a safe space for the individual. In this instance, the person with the shame bind is supported to "stay with self," to trust self through the emotions associated with the early childhood threatening experience — to breathe with trust in self, self-acceptance, self-support, and physically experience hope (lean forward into life) for a more confident and vibrant future.

Body Armor

The term "body armor" technically is not a Gestalt term, having been originally developed by Wilhelm Reich in his book "Character Analysis," but for me, this term communicates how shame binds are reflected in how we learn how to hold and use our body. Body armor is just that, a protective shield-like posture wherein we develop a physical holding of self that protects us from some imagined or actually experienced danger or trauma in life.

The experience of shame, for example, can become a permanent mind-body armor, not just how we think about or psychologically perceive our self as a result of some psychological trauma ala Stanley Keleman's book "Your Body Speaks Its Mind." The physical experience may be one of tensing, tightening certain body parts, holding one's breath, feeling lack of strength to support self in arms, legs, etc. Again, this experience of being rejected or shamed when we want to reach out in times of need is especially significant when it happens to us in childhood. In literally thousands of cases I have seen shame binds in youths, teens and adults that originated in childhood when as a child the person experienced situations such as constant angry and violent confrontations between parents, actual physical and sexual abuse toward the child, or the child being left alone without the care of a parent, etc.

These situations resulted in the development of an incomplete Gestalt or shame bind that sub-consciously led the person to doubt and pull back in shame when experiencing difficult life challenges, especially those where a person has to speak up, be seen, experiment with new behaviors, and generally express themselves with confidence in difficult situations. Again, the physical component that is a shame bind may be the inability to feel strength in one's arms, or energy to speak in one's throat, or strength in one's legs needed to take action necessary to support oneself in a challenging life situation.

Personally, my experiences as a Latino boy with a mama who could not teach me the cultural and social ways of the United States, led me to have a body armor of shying away from learning experiences wherein my self-esteem was threatened, e.g., where I could be laughed at or ridiculed by others for not knowing how to think, act, or feel in a particular situation. This, again for me, was especially strong in my early schooling experiences, when I did not always have a clear understanding or guidance with respect to how to act or make the most of my learning tasks. Rather than having a flexible physical body of confidence and eagerness in school, I had a posture or armor of hiding and not feeling strength (confidence) in my body that I could be effective and masterful in learning situations.

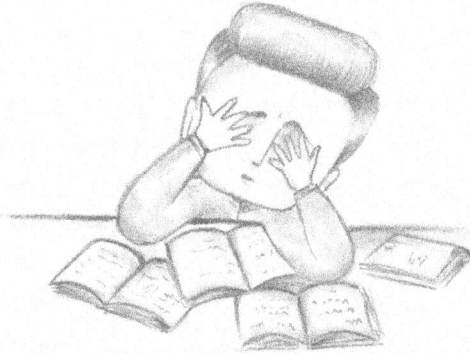

After sharing my challenging growth experiences in talks, including how Gestalt counseling work helped me develop greater psychological strength, I often ask audiences if they can connect a body feeling to experiences when they shy away from trusting themselves or acting confidently in a challenging life situation. Heads nod in affirmation: Yes, my body does or feels this or this. I continue with the following: "Get in touch with how your body feels in such situations, and stay with that feeling — accentuate the feeling, if you can . . . Now, can you associate an image of yourself as a child having a similar body feeling, and can you picture where you are, what is happening?" Many heads again nod in agreement.

This phenomenon shows how our body postures or armor "hold onto" our childhood experiences, and especially those where we experienced little or no "self-support," and primarily because of lack of "other support." The images we conjure up in such instances reflect "unfinished business," or sub-conscious memories of when we were unable to support ourselves to be effective in challenging situations. An interesting and fascinating extension of this phenomena is that often our visual images of past challenging situations are not always a direct image of our experience; rather, the mental representation that comes to our mind may be one that is symbolic or associated to visual images that were significant to us when we were children. The visual image that I have shared that I saw when initially getting in touch with my childhood experience of emotional chaos and abuse is the cartoon image showing a brawl between cartoon combatants.

My understanding of this image is that as a child I could not describe (experience the Gestalt Cycle of Experience) the experience of abuse in my family. However, I did associate the experience of abuse to the many cartoon fights that I watched. This association between cartoon fights and family situations of abuse were in my memory without words, and, initially, when I experienced a similar feeling of the "unfinished business" as an adult, I could only access the difficult childhood experiences indirectly through the cartoon image. To integrate the feelings and thoughts associated with this image, I had to stay with the difficult feelings until a new figural image emerged that allowed me to explore, experience, and experiment more deeply with the original experiences that were traumatic for me, when I was unable and did not know how to support myself. Little by little as an adult in counseling, I learned to support myself to work through the difficult feelings and related images from the "unfinished business" of my childhood.

The "Empty Chair Technique:" Integrating
Weakness and Strength and Building Self-Support

A primary strategy to develop self-support through Gestalt therapy, as well as how I've adapted it to Gestalt

Educational Counseling, is the use of the empty chair technique. This technique allows a person to directly experience key dynamics related to the process of personal growth, especially how we often develop splits in our self-process into two opposite and opposing positions, where at one end or pole we try to support our growth and at the other pole, we often mistrust or are negative toward supporting our efforts to change and grow psychologically (shame bind). Even worse, sometimes we have two negative poles, e.g., "I can't," where we doubt ourselves, and also criticize ourselves, "You're stupid!" Fritz Perls identified this polarity as our "Top Dog" and "Underdog." In the latter instance, a person experiences at one pole a negative, criticizing self and at the other end, an equally negative self-negating self.

Through the empty chair technique, a person acts out a dialogue between what Gestalt psychologists call "polarities" (two opposite positions). In one chair, let's say chair A, the person acts out doubts they may have toward a life challenge; changing chairs, the individual, now in chair B, responds to the position of the self in Chair A. The therapist, counselor, (Gestalt Educator) keenly pays attention to feelings, posture, musculature movements, voice, and words (our some*body*) that the person experiences when going back and forth in the chairs, and supports the individual to become more conscious of the dynamics of both positions to the point that there is a greater awareness of how the positions support or do not support personal growth (movement along the "Gestalt Cycle of Experience"). Persons are encouraged to experiment with alternative forms of acting and habitual ways of responding to their internal psychological conflicts.

In the book "Gestalt Is," Fritz Perls argues that most persons need to be re-sensitized and re-mobilized to get in touch with how they have separated from experiencing their true needs and wants. The aim of the empty chair technique is to support the development of greater awareness for how a person is stuck or how he or she is not supporting their unique growth needs. "Chair work," as it is called, truly is an emotional and awareness-building experience where a person, under the support of the therapist or counselor, learns to try out new ways of thinking, feeling, and behaving in service of uniting or integrating a self that accepts, honors, and lives out their uniqueness.

In a later chapter (Gestalt Educational Counseling) I will show how I have adapted the Gestalt empty chair technique into my work with community college students and ethnically diverse community members to create a one-session growth experience regarding how individuals can assume more self-support and personal responsibility for meeting life's challenges using a Gestalt perspective.

Doing Experiments to Test Out Different Gestalts

The Gestalt therapist or counselor helps clients become clear about how to address psychological challenges related to personal growth by helping persons "experiment" with alternative actions related to what they are experiencing and communicating by their emotions and musculature reactions, especially when a person is experiencing shame binds. Erving and Miriam Polster in their book "Gestalt Therapy Integrated," note that Gestalt personal development work goes beyond "aboutism" or talking about life and life's challenges; rather, Gestalt personal development methods rely on direct trial and error learning where the client focuses on how experiencing one's feelings lead to change and personal growth. Related to experiments, I have worked with thousands of college students, professionals, and community persons where they directly experience the terribleness of feeling hopeless and not supported, and then experience the action of truly feeling love toward self, even though such an action may never, literally, have been experienced by the person in their entire life! Truly, there have been countless times where I have heard the following phrase: "I never have loved myself!" This is in each and every instance a marvelous experience of individual growth where the person doing the work is changed for the better!

Building Awareness of One's Process of Forming Gestalts

The central concept of Gestalt Therapy/Personal Development work is to help persons develop awareness of the way they respond to life's daily challenges and emergencies. Another way of saying this is that Gestalt personal development work helps us become aware of our unique process for forming Gestalts in the effort to make sense of our existence, e.g., how we go about forming meaningful wholes in how we understand our lives. Each of us "is born unique," and we live a unique existence, and we develop personal themes for how we go about meeting our needs and wants. Unfortunately, either by the way we interpret life or from how our environment does or does not support us to express our uniqueness, each of us can develop processes or themes that do not support the expression of our uniqueness. Gestalt personal development work helps us to become aware of how we do or do not support the expression of our uniqueness.

For instance, a major theme that I have seen in many students of color in college is that they initially are doubtful and fearful of trusting and believing in their ability to master the challenges of college. They experience what is commonly known as "fear-of-failure," rather than "achievement motivation." The Gestalt work I do with students helps them learn about where their fears and doubts originate as well as how to support themselves to get beyond their fears and doubts to develop their inner strength and confidence to take on the responsibility of learning at a high level and succeeding in their individual academic pursuits.

The Concepts of Figure/Ground and
Becoming Aware of Gestalt Formation

One of the most powerful ideas that I have learned from Gestalt psychotherapy is the idea of "figure/ground." Originally coming from Gestalt perceptual psychology, research discovered that when persons perceive or experience their environment, what stands out in their perception is the most prominent feature of the environment (figure), and what is not so important to perception remains in the background (ground), e.g., a terrifying fire becomes figure versus a beautiful sunset, which becomes ground. Gestalt psychologists also discovered that perception is influenced by individual motivation in that what a person is motivated toward achieving influences what is focused on with regard to perception. For instance, a person who is hungry will see food-related stimuli more prominently in the environment; similarly, if a person is motivated toward competition, competitive situations will be seen as more prominent in the environment.

Gestalt therapists extended the terms figure/ground to describe psychological experiences, where what is most prominent psychologically in a person's experience stands out (figure), with phenomena not so central in the background (ground). The interesting point is that often the background phenomena is more important for a person's psychological growth and development than what initially stands out (figure) as the most prominent psychological perception. A basic example that I have seen over and over is that for persons experiencing anxiety the physical sensations are most often prominent, and what stands out usually are the tensions and nervousness of the body. However, in the background or ground of this experience lie the origin for the why of the anxiety (the previous experience of frustration of needs and wants) as well as possible options for resolving the anxiety.

In the background are the original learning experiences that were too difficult to face and handle effectively. These experiences were driven to the background or subconscious of our awareness because the original fearful and threatening experiences were too frightening to be experienced and resolved (progressing through the Gestalt Cycle of Experience). Needless to say, these unsolved background experiences, again, called "unfinished business" by Gestalt therapists, become part of the background for how a person responds to life's challenges.

Gestalt counseling methods help a person become aware of the background (ground) of the original experience for anxiety and other psychological experiences, and, importantly, help a person to learn to use their psychological and perceptual processes in a clear way to distinguish what is most important or figural in support of personal development, versus what is not so central to meeting the psychological growth needs of the person. Being able to be aware

and distinguish between what challenges are most important in life rather than being controlled by unfinished anxieties from the past is important work for Gestalt therapists,
as well as helping persons become aware of what personal
strength individuals have with regard to effectively facing
psychological challenges.

"Staying With" Difficult Sensations Until
We Develop Gestalts of Self-support

From building awareness for how persons are feeling/
behaving in their body related to psychological conflicts,
Gestalt personal development work supports persons to
broaden their awareness of physical feelings and actions by
"staying with" these sensations until a clearer picture (figure) emerges of what is behind or is "the ground" of a person's feelings and bodily reactions. This "staying with"
difficult sensations can lead to a person supporting their natural ability (organismic self-regulation) to effectively act to
resolve difficult challenges. For example, rapid breathing or
tension in the throat may initially be experienced as frightening; however, staying with these feelings may lead to
awareness that they signal the need to express different
emotions and thoughts, such as anger or, even love, that is
hidden behind the experience of tension and anxiety.

Staying with feelings/sensations leads to the emergence
of a clearer "figure" as to what a person's body, organism is
communicating related to psychological conflicts stemming
from unfulfilled or unfinished needs and wants. In the end,
staying with difficult emotions means staying with one's
unique self as we work at learning to face and live life as we
want. An example can be useful here. One of the big fears

that persons express to me when I do Gestalt work with them is the desire to not want to cry. Nevertheless, in all instances, crying leads to becoming conscious and aware of some part of ourselves that is not being responded to or acknowledged with respect to the need for love and acceptance and support. Staying with self through the fear of crying and to the actual experience of crying often results in experiencing our real needs for love, acceptance, and support.

The Gestalt of Completing I: Experiencing *CONTACT* with My Developing/Learning Self

When personal experiments lead to more clarity about who one is and how one may want to develop psychologically and live life, we experience "contact" with our unique self. I can describe "contact" as the experience of reintegration of one's self (thinking, feeling, and behaving) so that the self is different than before the growth experience, i.e., there is a different or new experience of self. In his book "The Creative Process in Gestalt Therapy," Dr. Joseph Zinker writes of persons having a "posture for being in the world" and that "the most profound discoveries or learnings take place when a person is self-directed . . . when he (she) supports self . . . and when his (her) total sensorimotor organism participates in formation of figure-ground." This, for me, is "contact" according to Gestalt personal development work. Contact is when we as unique persons experience the process of having a felt ownership for who we are, our true "Learning Self." It is a beautiful experience!

**Unfinished Gestalts are "Unfinished Business"
vis-a-vis the Development of Our Unique Self**

Finally, the Gestalt concept of "unfinished business" points to aspects of the experience of one's psychological growth that are unfinished or incomplete. From birth to death, we have experiences that challenge us to develop, change, and be more complete as a person who can adapt to life in an effective manner. When challenging experiences are not completed in a manner that result in being more complete in our ability to trust and be responsible for achieving our growth and satisfying our needs and wants, we are left with "unfinished business." Using the Gestalt Cycle of Experience as a guide and Gestalt personal development methods such as the empty chair technique to progressively build more self-support, assists us to move through each of our unique unfinished business so we can progressively become more capable and self-directing human beings.

Summary and Thoughts about Chapter 2

In conclusion to this introduction to Gestalt personal development concepts, I want to put forward an argument that these concepts are effective in helping us grow psychologically because they reflect and explicate what is effective versus non-effective living. In short, what is special about our experience of being human is our ability to be aware or conscious of ourselves, as well as to use our awareness to take actions that lead us to be effective and satisfied with life, i.e., grow and develop as a unique person. In this regard, throughout our life we can both support or hinder our ability to be aware and effective in meeting our individual "needs and wants." When we learn through negative life experiences, especially in childhood, to limit our ability to use our personal awareness to take effective action, we limit our effectiveness to be who we are and how we want to live.

Negative life experiences create psychological conflicts within us that we can either continue to live with or choose to change so as to learn to grow past these conflicts. I describe this challenge in the following way: Our future will be our past, or we can bring our past into our present, and choose a new future! I have found for myself and many others that using Gestalt personal development methods to move through the Gestalt Cycle of Experience helps re-do and create a more powerful "Learning Self" that helps us undo what we have learned in life that lessens and gets in the way of our psychological effectiveness and completeness as persons.

Chapter 3

The Gestalt Concept of Figure/GROUND:
My Childhood Legacy is Formed

First, note how in the title of this chapter I have capitalized the term GROUND. I do this to emphasize that I am going to focus on how our childhood experiences often are background or ground to our adult psychological existence. As such, in this chapter I share how my childhood experiences framed my adult personality. In my childhood, I learned to think about myself and develop habits of being that directed my thinking, feeling, and behaving. Although I did not know it in my youth, I would have to become aware and let go of my "Childhood Legacy" in order to free myself to live my uniqueness and work toward achieving completeness as a person.

First, let's do a quick review of the Gestalt concept of Figure/Ground. In any perception, *figure* is what is most prominent and stands out in our perception, with *ground* being what is in the background of the figure, which is usually not as prominent in our perception. For example, if in our place of residence there is a fire, the fire is figure, and the sandwich we were about to eat becomes ground, or what is not the primary focus in our perception. Once we clear ourselves from the threat of the fire, the hunger for the sandwich may become figure once again. This same principle applies to our psychological life. In our perception of the world, what is figure is what is most important to us psychologically, but in the background are aspects of the figure that are important that can make the perception more complete, whole.

For example, if I am a person who is not confident about

speaking in front of groups (for which the majority of persons in the U.S. identify as their greatest fear), the thoughts and resulting physical experience of anxiety (sweaty hands, shaky legs, dizziness, etc.) is figure, and the actual content of the talk is the ground, which is not as prominent as the experienced negative emotions. Our life is a series of figure/ground experiences which we build up in our memory, and which progressively create what Hanson and Mendius in their book "Buddha's Brain: The Practical Neuroscience of Happiness, Love, and Wisdom" call the "horizons of our perception." These perceptions color how we approach life; that is, they become figural or more important for us in how we perceive and react to life, both positively or negatively. In this chapter, I look at my experiences in childhood, which were *figure* for me at the time of their occurrence, but which have become ground for my adult psychological life, often containing fear, doubt, and shame that lessen my adult ability to handle life effectively.

"Everybody is born unique . . ." This is a quote I noted earlier in this book, which I use to commence motivational speeches. Using this quote is my way to capture the motivational attention of listeners (just as with you) to look at themselves critically with respect to their unique needs, wants, and attempts at achieving personal growth. Again, without fail, people hearing this quote all raise their hands in agreement. "Yes, we are all born unique!"

"But, again, there's more," I share. "Everybody is born unique... but most of us die copies!" To this, again, there is generally a gasp and a resigned raising of hands in agreement from the majority of the audience.

I go on with the following question: "Will those who want to die a copy, raise their hand." Always again, without fail, no one raises their hand! I continue, "If most of us agree that everyone is born unique, and also that most of us die copies, then why doesn't anyone want to die a copy? And, if no one wants to die a copy, why do so many of us end our lives as copies?" There is hesitancy to answer this question, but, generally, the reasons given for why most of us die copies, that is, acting not from one's center but from how we think we should behave to fit in to the world around us, is because we tend to follow the lead of others, or because too many of us find it too difficult to express our uniqueness.

I press on to probe for a main reason why many of us may find it hard to become aware of and express our uniqueness. I give a hint: "Think of a four-letter word that may explain why we die copies instead of being our individual uniqueness." Every time I provide the hint, the answer soon rings out: "Fear!" Yes, yes, yes — fear! But what does this have to do with the title of this chapter, "My Childhood Legacy," and the concept of figure/ground? Did my legacy lead me to become a copy? Or did my Childhood Legacy help me learn to be true to my individual uniqueness? And what does fear have to do with all of this? And what is this legacy I talk about, anyway? And what does all this have to do with my/your perception of self and the world and our personal and professional development? Let me press on to give my answers to these questions.

My Childhood Legacy is my childhood experiences that shaped the person I have become, and created the "horizons of my perception." In my childhood lies much of the answer (the ground) for how I have learned to perceive the world and to support or not support myself psychologically to express my uniqueness as a human being. But the answer to how my childhood relates to the expression of my unique-ness and my personal and professional development does not simply lie in understanding how my early years explain my hesitancy toward or lack of achievement of personal growth. Rather, it is in re-experiencing and re-doing of my childhood, especially through the use of Gestalt personal development methods, where I have found the answer to how to learn to support myself to express my unique self.

Also, this understanding has helped me to help many others to step into and "lean forward into life!" (thanks again Abe Levitsky for sharing this phrase!) on the path to honoring and becoming their unique selves. In this regard, there is a quote of mine that expresses how re-experiencing my childhood has helped me develop my uniqueness and supported my personal and professional growth: "Our fu-ture will be our past, unless we can bring our past into our present, and choose our future!" This quote is the core of how I have learned to have greater awareness of myself, as well as helping me develop the competence to counsel oth-ers to understand and support their individual uniqueness and personal growth. Gestalt personal development theory, in turn, has been the driving force that has helped me "bring my past into the present and choose my future!"

I will continue referring to my motivational speeches to explain how I learned to "Know, Understand, Feel, Choose, and Act" (*Saber, Entender, Sentir, Escoger, y Hacer*) my uniqueness, as well as how coming to an understand-ing of my Childhood Legacy led me to be more effective at developing my uniqueness, and by extension, supporting my personal and professional development. And, impor-tantly, I will connect my ideas to the experience and ex-pression of fear, because I have learned that fear is the biggest psychological roadblock to expressing our unique self. So, let's not wait any longer about defining this childhood legacy of mine, as well as learning how over time I have brought my legacy forward into my present so as to be able to support the expression of my unique personal and professional development.

In my speeches, I share my childhood experiences as a way of getting audiences to understand my message about how to use Gestalt personal development concepts to support clarifying and supporting the growth of one's personal uniqueness. I do this because without qualification I know that it is my work in Gestalt that has freed me to be clearer about who I am and express myself appropriate to myself. In my speeches, I communicate how my legacy from childhood initially served to move me toward being a copy, and to not support my personal development to becoming my unique self.

One such anecdote that I share is that in great part because of my past learning of lack of self-support I flunked out at my first attempt to attend college, which I did at Laney College in Oakland, California. In this experience, I was a copy of a person who wasn't clear about how college can help one choose and develop their unique self. Rather than resolving my fear about speaking up in college and focusing on learning, I spent most of my time avoiding learning by playing around, chasing girls, playing basketball, and generally giving in to my need for obtaining pleasure. The "figures" of my life revolved around gaining sensual pleasures, rather than focusing on developing my unique strengths as a person. But let's go back to my early childhood to see how I began learning not to support myself to think, feel, and act my true self.

One of my favorite personal stories related to my Child-hood Legacy of fear has to do with my early experiences with my abusive father (I cannot separate the word abusive from father when referring to my father, even when I take a calming deep breath . . . this means more work or "unfin-ished business" still to be done). This is the story: I remem-ber being held underwater at the top of my head for what seemed like an interminably long time by my angry father at Fleishhacker Pool at Ocean Beach in San Francisco, Cali-fornia. I remember thinking, feeling I was going to die. I was seven, and I really believed I was going to die, that my father was going to kill me.

When I share this story, I ask audiences what they think I was feeling at that moment. They often respond with what they imagine I was *thinking,* not what I was feeling in my body. "You thought your father was going to kill you; you thought you were going to die; you thought . . ." I ask them for feelings I may have had. They warm up to it. "You felt hopeless, powerless, lost, alone . . ."

"Yes, yes, I must have! But still, hopeless, lost, and alone are thoughts" I answer. "For example, I think, 'I have no hope at this moment; no one is here to help me.'

"But," I continue to ask, "What are the physical feelings associated with these thoughts? What was happening in my body?"

Here is where participants dig a little deeper. "Hopeless-ness," they share, "can feel like lack of strength and/or ten-sion in the shoulders, loss of breath, dizziness, etc. Thinking "I'm alone" can result in feelings like "tears welling up in the eyes, losing all energy in my arms and legs, going blank in the mind."

In this initial analysis of an early childhood experience

of mine lies one of the core tenets for me for what it means to do Gestalt personal growth work. Feelings, what one experiences in one's body, are what is important, versus just thinking. Feelings are important because our legacy from childhood lies mostly in subconscious memory of emotions that have been stored in the musculature of our body. That is, what lessens our ability to act freely (in Spanish, "*con voluntad*") is bound-up physical energy in our body that stops us from supporting ourselves to act in ways that express our uniqueness. (Again, these physical-psychological blocks are called shame binds, of which I will address more in depth later). Now, I want to take a short detour to better understand this point about feeling versus thinking.

In the fall semester of 2018, in my "Introduction to Psychology" class, I came to a deeper understanding as to the impact of feeling versus thinking with regard to our ability to be autonomous and self-directing (take more ownership) in our experience of our thoughts, feelings, and actions — to act our unique selves. In childhood, which is our most psychologically vulnerable time of life, our brain is undergoing continual development, and the emotional part of the brain, the amygdala, is more powerful than the reasoning part of the brain, the pre-frontal cortex (PFC). As a result, we are more likely to experience emotional and related physical associations rather than cognitive reasoning experiences.

However, the explanation of this process is literally a little more involved than this! What I learned in that 2018 semester is that our childhood learning lies deeper in our physiology than our new brain, the PFC, or the middle part of our brain, the amygdala. Our childhood learning, mostly what is called associational reflex learning, happens in a more ancient part of our physiology, the cerebellum, or our "old brain." Here, when we are threatened, similar to my experience of threat at being held underwater at Fleishhacker Pool, our learning happens when neurotransmitters in our cerebellum, an ancient brain (that even fish, birds, and other animals possess) develop memory associations connected to our body's reflexive reaction to being threatened, and the learning is more basic than thinking about what is happening to us.

The learning that we do is called "procedural learning," and involves our specific physiological reactions to the threat as experienced in our body. Much like animals who also have our ancient brain, we learn to associate "body feelings" of threat to the danger we experience, and this learning, much like animals, is not so much a learning involving rational or logical thinking. Rather, it is a learning in our body, where we tense and release stress-related neurons that activates our hypothalamus and sympathetic nervous system and move us toward what is known as fight or flight.

So, the short of it is that my feeling self was mostly in charge when I was seven, and so my legacy was more one of learning, mostly subconscious, feelings and associated body sensations of threat, fear, doubt, etc., versus learning to have reasoned thoughts about what I was experiencing as a little boy! I would carry these subconscious body-experienced emotions into my adult thinking and acting more than reasoned thoughts about what I experienced as a little boy.

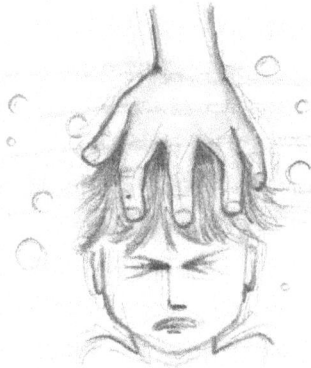

Let me slow down and take a close look at the above drawing. Can you imagine what thoughts I was having as a child who had not developed his capacity to have reason? Not too much complicated thinking, huh? But can you imagine what I physically was experiencing in my shoulders, mouth, eyes, and throat? I can. My shoulders? Tightness, tension. My mouth? Tightness, and again, pressure. Eyes? Tension, tightness. Emotions? Fear, anger, hurt, sadness, disgust, threat. These non-cognitive physical reactions and associations were "figure" for me at the time and are what became part of my memory, and, as such, these physical sensations are what I needed to become aware of and experience directly when I did my psychological work as an adult! I would have to face and unpack or differentiate my chaotic cartoon image of my Childhood Legacy!

I want to now continue with how I share myself with others so as to help them trust me and open up and be willing to do work to be more aware, know themselves better, and therefore begin to more effectively take charge of their personal growth. I have learned both from reading and my direct teaching and group work with people that opening up and sharing myself supports others to open up about their doubts, fears, etc. Some books that I'm familiar with and have used in classes related to this process are: "Why Am I Afraid to Tell You Who I Am? by John Joseph Powell, "Psychotherapy: The Purchase of Friendship" by William Schofield, "Joy" by William Schutz, and "Person to Person" by Carl Rogers.

The following is how I open up and share myself with others. I write down the childhood experience, e.g., Fleishhacker Pool, and review the feelings and associated thoughts that go with my experience: *Feelings*: lack of strength in my shoulders; tension in my shoulders; loss of breath; dizziness; losing strength in my limbs; mind going blank, tears welling up in my eyes, etc. *Thoughts*: "I am hopeless; I have no one to turn to; my father hates me; I am no good, etc." This is my "legacy list." This is the list of what my body carried forward into my future life experiences, as well as how my mind may have subconsciously interpreted what my body experienced. (This has proven interesting to me because my mind at that time made subconscious associations based on what I had experienced up to that point in my life, e.g., cartoons, fantasies, incomplete memories, etc. More of this to come.)

The above list of my feelings is a list of how my body and child brain (directed in great part by my "old brain," the cerebellum) might have reacted to real or imagined threats to me from the outside world. An important point here is that in adulthood I brought my childhood emotional experiences, much of it from my subconscious, to my present experiences, which means that my childhood self, including emotions and thoughts, is what I often used in the present to respond to psychological challenges I experienced in everyday life as an adult. And, I have learned that for me, unless I reexperience this past directly in the present and support myself to face the emotional binds that are part of my body's memory/legacy of my past, the past will continue to direct me away from supporting myself to act in a unique way that is directed by my adult reasoning self rather than by my fearful, emotional child self!

Another experience that I share when I give talks, recounts when my brother and I had to go to live at St. Vincent's School for Boys in San Rafael, California. At the age of seven, following a fearful experience of hiding for two weeks from my father in a house in North Oakland, my mother went to work as a live-in maid with a family in Oakland, and my brother and I had to go to live at St. Vincent's School for Boys, a facility for children from broken homes. The story I tell is of the first night at St. Vincent's when I was placed in one dorm and separated from my eleven-month older brother, Frank, who was put in a different dorm. My brother recounts that around two o'clock in the morning, I showed up at the side of his bed rubbing my eyes and crying, *"Yo quiero mama!"*

The thoughts that audiences say I must have had were the following: hopelessness (*desesperado*); abandonment (*abandonado*); rejection; confusion about how my life would turn out; anger and hate toward my father; being lost and confused. The body feelings associated with the latter thoughts that audiences come up with are the following: dizziness; tension in my arms, neck, back, and legs; shortness of breath; furrowed brow; the muscles around my eyes causing the shedding of tears, etc. Again, all of the latter thoughts and feelings are part of my Childhood Legacy list.

This list makes up in great part how my thinking and related body sensations from childhood have led to the fig-ure-grounds of my experiences in adulthood. This legacy list defines in great part the perceived limitations and pos-sibilities, both conscious and subconscious, I have in my mind-body (organism) for defining myself and choosing ac-tions to direct myself in life as an adult. Gestalt personal de-velopment work has helped me increase my awareness of how my Childhood Legacy directs my present, and has al-lowed me to develop my abilities to stop being directed by my past ineffective emotional learning (see "The Handbook of Higher Consciousness" by Ken Keyes and "Games People Play" by Eric Berne for similar texts on how learned child-hood "emotional addictions" or "emotional tapes" influence adult behavior).

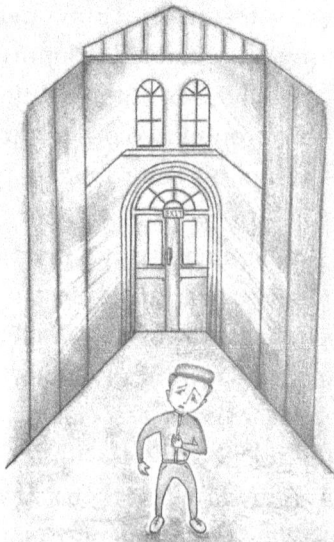

Lost and confused at Grant School

One more significant personal story that I share in talks is when I was a second grader, having recently returned to the United States after having lived in Costa Rica for a year-and-a-half. I had forgotten how to speak English. The story involves me seeing myself as a little boy standing in a hallway at Grant School on 29th Street in Oakland, California. The little boy is seemingly confused and lost (I went to eleven different schools from kindergarten through high school). The thoughts others think I must have had were the following: "Who am I? Why am I here? What do I do? Should I run away? Where do I go? Who can help me? I don't know what to do nor who to turn to for help." (An interesting side thought here is that my thinking was in Spanish because I had forgotten English). The body feelings associated with the latter thoughts may have been one or all of the following: tension in my forehead and welling up of tears in my eyes; shortness of breath; tension in my shoulders; tightness and nervousness in my legs; confusion in my mind, etc. Can you see that my Childhood Legacy list continued to grow? Can you imagine how this Childhood Legacy list negatively influenced my ability to support myself to express and become my unique self in school, social and work situations, etc.? For example, how my Childhood Legacy list affected my attending and flunking out of Laney College in 1967?

Again, Rick Hanson and Richard Mendius in their book "Buddha's Brain," note that difficult experiences in childhood can color the landscape of our brain with negative thoughts and emotions that, in turn, become the lens through which we learn to perceive and interpret the paths and horizons of our life's experiences. For me, my early childhood experiences, while having much love from my mother and brother, was filled with much fear, doubt, hurt, anger, confusion, etc., stemming from the way my father treated me and my brother and mother. This colored and framed the landscape of my developing brain, which I relied on in my childhood experiences, and would continue to rely on in my future to understand, negotiate, and navigate my life's challenges; importantly, my difficult and hurtful experiences became locked deep in my mind and body — in my cerebellum's confusing physical associations of childhood bodily feelings connected with potential threats to my well-being.

This was my legacy from childhood. This legacy would unfold more and more throughout my childhood, adolescence, and young adulthood as I, in retrospect, now see as halting efforts, first, to find my real or unique self, and second, to support my real self to breathe strength, passion, courage, and joy into my existence. My road to personal and professional development too often was filled with tenuous breath and non-supporting bodily sensations as I haltingly moved to support ownership and expression of my unique existence.

Chapter 4

The Gestalt Concept of FIGURE/Ground: With Gestalt Work I Begin to Clarify the Impact of My Childhood Legacy on the Expression of My Unique Self

In this chapter, I connect how my Childhood Legacy defined my awareness and knowledge of myself as an adult, in many ways undermining my ability to be aware of how I did or did not support expression of my unique self. My recollection of my childhood is that I often went against how I wanted to see myself and how I wanted to act. Specifically, key negative events in my childhood colored my perception of myself in the world and affected how I thought, felt, and acted, and so my ability to be my unique self was limited by my inability to understand and free myself from the doubts and fears I learned in my formative years. My challenge in adulthood was to get to know myself, and to learn how to liberate myself from the negative learning of my youth that hampered me in adulthood-my Childhood Legacy.

I continue into my adulthood . . . At about the age of thirty-two, I began to become more keenly aware and develop a clearer "figure" out of the "ground" of my Childhood Legacy; here I started to steadily unfold the possibilities of my unique being by increasing my ability to understand and experiment with new ways of being, rather than being directed by what Ken Keyes in his book "Handbook of Higher Consciousness" calls "security, sensation, and power addictions." I started to realize that my life involved choice: Choice about what to think, choice about what to feel, and choice about how to act. My greater awareness of myself and of ways to enhance my expressiveness as a unique person developed in great part because of my introduction to Gestalt personal development work.

This first happened while I was attending the University of Minnesota in Minneapolis, Minnesota. I was in the middle of my doctoral program in Counseling and Student Personnel Psychology, and I was searching for a way to support myself through all the anxieties that resulted from doing a doctorate — my imagined fear of being rejected by my doctoral committee, and more extensively, being rejected by the world, and the doubt of whether I would make it as a psychologist. Or, at the other extreme, would I end up in the gutter or back on welfare like in my childhood, and the fear that I would not be able to continue having my beautiful little family.

The latter were my "thinking" or cognitive fears and doubts, and they were supported by my physiological fears or "body emotions" developed in childhood: tightness in the muscles in my legs; holding my breath; dizziness; tension in my arms, neck, and back, etc. At the time I was trying to do my doctorate, my existence included trying to help raise four beautiful children with a partner who kept challenging me to finish my doctorate, as well as challenging what in retrospect I understand is part of my unique identity as a Latino person in development in the U.S.A.— that is, to be of service to my Latin@ community and the poor.

After unsuccessfully trying a number of therapists to help me with my anxiety for how to understand and be me, I enrolled in a graduate course in the Social Work Department at the University of Minnesota with Dr. Bart Grossman — Introduction to Gestalt Therapy. Wow, wow, wow! Really, I mean wow, wow, wow! Including reading about the theory and methods of Gestalt therapy, this course was an experiential journey into the students' psychological life journeys from a Gestalt perspective.

Each week the professor did what I experienced as very scary body-mind awareness Gestalt work to help us directly experience and work on our fears, doubts, hidden emotions, and hopes for personal growth. In the fifth week, after a month-and-a-half of desperately wanting to stand and speak up, I dared to raise my hand and say, "I want to work!" Wow, wow, wow, again! Dr. Grossman asked me to stand (we, some thirty-five of us, were on the carpet and pillows on the floor). I stood. Dr. Grossman said, "Tell me about yourself?" I took in a big breath (which now many years later many students and others in the San Francisco-Oakland Bay Area and across our nation have done with me), and I blurted out what I can only call a "statement of would-be strength."

"I am one bad-ass MF. I am going to challenge our nation to make things right for people of color, cut out the bullshit, and help the poor be strong!"

Professor Grossman looked at me with a steely, steady gaze, and said: "I can see that you have a lot of tension in your legs, that you're standing almost only on the balls of your feet. Can you show me the other side of what you just shared?"

The other side? What? Here tears well up in my eyes as I recall the shock I felt at this request to show my weakness, rather than my facade of strength which had carried me halfway through my life and into my challenging doctoral studies (I think about a statistic that says that only 30 percent of doctoral candidates complete their doctorate ["all-but-dissertation"], and I think about the possibility that the reason so many of us don't make it through is because the

strength that we have to do so is at the most superficial —
but this is another book, article, talk, maybe).

I became dizzy at Dr. Grossman's question. I literally
started to dissociate or separate from my experience of myself in the moment. I felt as if I was suddenly far away from
the classroom situation. I was scared. Dr. Grossman's competence brought me back to the present. He, like I have now
learned to do as I work with others, looked into my eyes,
and connected me to him. I started to cry, and did so for a
long time. He watched my body, waited for me to move out
of my tear state, waiting for a new figure to emerge into
what I now know as a new "emergency," or emerging
Gestalt — a new figure coming out of the background of my
life experiences, and primarily from my Childhood Legacy.

Dr. Grossman asked me what I was experiencing. I told
him I felt tension in my hands. He asked me, "What do you
need? what do you want?" I looked at him with confusion.
Again, my experience was like that of so many others who
have since done Gestalt work with me. My hands out of
nowhere formed what to Dr. Grossman looked like the
emerging figure of a fist. "Do you need, want to hit something?" he asked. The feeling in my fists became stronger,
more pronounced. The energy in my arms became more
complete, figural. Dr. Grossman put up his hands, and for
what seemed like hours, but really was only about thirty
minutes, I hit and hit, and hit his open hands.

During this "work," I connected the violent outburst to
the hate and rage I held within me toward what I remember
as "my monster father." I recall that I became fearful that I
would break Dr. Grossman's hands. At one point, he looked
deep into my eyes (into my hidden subconscious psyche,
my Childhood Legacy) and asked me if I was okay. I looked

at him with a childlike sense of hope, and, said, "Yes!" We continued until I expended, for that moment at least, the energy associated with my deep anger and hate toward my father. My tears lessened. I felt lighter, less tense (*deshaugado* is what many of my Latin@ clients communicate to me after they do their Childhood Legacy work). My legs, though shaky, felt stronger and steadier, more peaceful, and soft. We finished. Wow, wow, wow! My first real Gestalt work!

After class, I had a free moment with Dr. Grossman, and I sheepishly asked him what he thought of my work. "Was it good? Was the work of significance?" He answered, "It's a good beginning." "That sounds okay," I thought. "But what does it mean?" Let me continue to make sense of this for you, as I had to do for myself in my life.

As a contrast to Gestalt personal development work, I want to share a relevant piece of psychological work that I did before I started my doctoral studies. Although this work was psychodynamic (how different forces in my mind create the dynamic self-perceptions of me being me) and not Gestalt-focused work, I see it as important to understand the future Gestalt work that I would do that would indeed unlock my hidden Childhood Legacy and my potential to be my unique self. I had applied, with the help of a very special professor and friend from San Francisco State University's Master's Program in Counseling, Dr. Robert "Bob" Chope, and been accepted to the doctoral program in Counseling and Student Personnel Psychology at the University of Minnesota, Minneapolis. Receiving my letter of acceptance was a surreal experience because I did not in fact know to what I was headed. Nevertheless, as with most of my life experiences up to that point, I moved forward with hope that I could handle the challenge. This was until about two weeks before beginning my drive to Minnesota with my family of four: Anita, Jake, Maria-Elena, and Teresita (Tita).

At the threshold of leaving for the University of Minnesota, I began to have a continuous series of nightmares that truly shook my confidence about beginning doctoral study. The nightmares went on for days, and involved me being in a pitch-black house, and being chased by a monster who was trying to catch me.

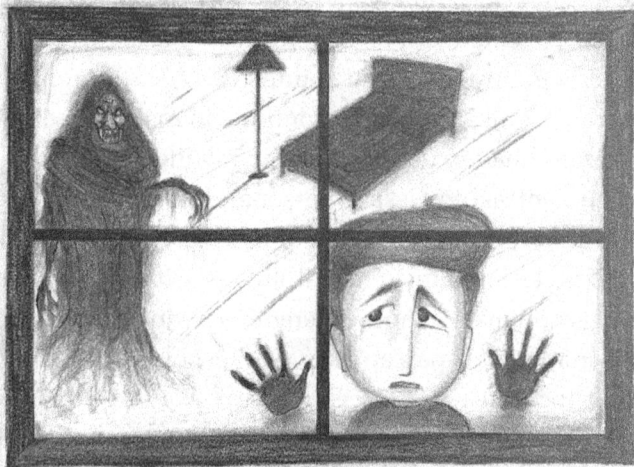

My fear in the dream was overwhelming. Every step I took to run away from the monster, steps that were hampered by dreamlike slow movement, were filled with unimaginable terror. My body was extremely tense in my dream, yet in some way I moved through the house trying to find a window by which to escape the monster. Every window I came to was bolted shut! My terror was palpable (I could feel it throughout my body, and I'm sure it was made up of all the bodily feelings I had built up in my Childhood Legacy. Remember Little Mario who was held under water by his father, being separated from his brother at St. Vincent's School for Boys; hiding in my desk behind other students in my elementary school classes?)

Finally, I came to an open window, and as I began to step hopefully through the window, the monster snatched me! Each and every night for a week, the dream continued with the same terrifying ending. Although I woke from the dream, I would return to it when and if I fell asleep. I was so terrified in the dream that I slept very little each night. Finally, exhausted, I made an appointment with a psychiatrist, Dr. Robert Dolgoff of the Berkeley Family Therapy Institute, a counseling center that I previously went to for marital counseling.

Dr. Dolgoff listened to the recounting of my dreams, and then asked me to tell him a little about my life. Crying, I shared the difficulties that my mother, brother, and I had experienced with my father. One story that I shared was of a situation that I had experienced as a child before having to go to St. Vincent's School for Boys. Fearful of the effect that my father's violent ugliness could have on her children, my mother took my brother and me away from my father one night, and we hid out at a house in North Oakland (I stop now to experience the strong emotion of wondering whether I ever truly thanked my Latina, mono-lingual, Spanish-speaking mama for how she sacrificed to save my brother and me from the ugliness of my father).

Back to my meeting with Dr. Dolgoff. The central aspect of this *"pesadilla,"* that was very vivid for me, was that my mother warned my brother and me not to go near the windows (*no vayan por las ventanas!*), which were closed off by vinyl roller shades. I shared this story with little awareness or insight and with little understanding of its relationship to my present life. At the end, Dr. Dolgoff leaned toward me and asked, "Could that house where you hid as a child be the house in your dreams, and could that monster be your father?" I stared at him and started to cry with great intensity, which I did without stopping for about a half an hour. After this session with Dr. Dolgoff, the nightmares stopped, and I went off to Minnesota in my four-door, ocean-steel-blue Pontiac Ventura with my little family, not expecting that my journey would take me into many more fearful experiences that would require increasingly more challenging efforts on my part to clarify and become aware of how my Childhood Legacy was relevant to my day-to-day efforts to define and be the self I wanted to be.

Not all growth is about Gestalt Work: "Other Support" is huge!

As witnessed above, not everything about my personal development, as Dr. Abe Levitsky would say to me in later years in our therapy sessions, was related to Gestalt work. And yes, I agree that a good portion of my psychological growth is about the help, guidance and "other support" I received along the way from loving people who supported me to face difficult life challenges. However, the "core" of my personal development breakthrough came from my Gestalt work.

Continuing, I want to share two more non-Gestalt experiences as a contrast for understanding how Gestalt personal development work has more definitively provided me with the psychological strength and courage to be myself. One story was the moment when I was close to taking my preliminary oral exam wherein my committee of four PhDs could ask me anything about my doctoral courses of study and the focus of my dissertation, which was about how to improve the motivation and success of underrepresented and underprepared minority students in college (helping the less fortunate that my mother had instilled in me as being important for my life).

After completing my first two years of doctoral coursework, I took an extra year to gain the courage to take and pass my four-hour statistics exam, which I did with a surprisingly good score. Now I had to move on to my oral preliminary examination where I would have to write a doctoral proposal, as well as meet for two hours with my doctoral committee when they could ask me anything about counseling psychology theory and practice, as well as specifics of what I intended to do for my dissertation research. And, one possibility was that they could fail me. I was terrified!

In preparation, I read what seemed like tons of literature and research on achievement motivation, generally, and, more specifically, about the achievement motivation of ethnically diverse underrepresented and underprepared students in college. My brain was literally oversaturated with information to the point of creating confusion for me, as well as increasing my anxiety whenever I tried to access my knowledge. In retrospect, my body was tense with my present challenge, but unbeknownst to me, also tense with the connections to my Childhood Legacy of fear and doubt. I now know that if I had done Gestalt work with this lack of self-support within me, I would have surely moved forward with more strength to finish my dissertation. I would have reflected on what I had previously learned and I then would have organized my knowledge to support my confidence to meet the challenge of my oral preliminary examination. However, this was not the case.

One evening, while studying in preparation for my preliminary oral exam, I had what I now think was a panic attack. I froze in fear and could not move! Somehow, I called a colleague of mine who was also in the same doctoral program, Leroy Gardner. Leroy, who formerly played center for the University of Minnesota basketball team, and even had played against the great Lew Alcindor, had become a dear friend of mine. We both worked in the Martin Luther King Jr. undergraduate Academic Advising office in the College of Liberal Arts at the University of Minnesota. Over the phone, I cried to Leroy that I was scared that I was going to fail in my doctorate, lose my family (my wife was threatening to divorce me if I didn't finish my doctorate), and that I felt lost and didn't know what to do.

Leroy came right over. With his six-foot, eight-inch frame, Leroy picked me up and walked me around my block. I can clearly see the neighborhood and the cold dark snowy Minnesota night, and Leroy providing me his loving strength (thank you, Leroy!). He told me over and over how special I was and how he and all the staff and students in the MLK program believed in me.

I want to share a funny and heartwarming story related to this anecdote. Years later when I was giving the keynote address at a National Academic Advising Association conference in San Diego, California, I recounted this story to the audience, and lo and behold, who stood up and called out, "And, that's the truth because I am Leroy Gardner!" Back to my story.

With Leroy's support, I continued my life journey, albeit

with doubt and trepidation, but truly I did not connect the outstanding FIGURE of my then-present emergency of approaching my preliminary oral exam to the GROUND of my Childhood Legacy, a legacy which filled my "body" with doubt and shame rather than confidence and high self-esteem. This awareness and clarity of perception about the connection between my Childhood Legacy and my adult self would happen many years later as I did more in-depth Gestalt personal development work.

One other experience I want to share that involves "other support" and non-Gestalt work, is the help I received from Dr. Thomas Skovholt, my dissertation advisor at the University of Minnesota. I share this experience for two reasons. The first reason is that life's successes for most of us involve support from others, and the second reason is that everyone is in the process of development, and this development is not all strictly psychological; part of our development is social, interpersonal, and cognitive. In graduate school, part of my developmental challenge had to do with my need to improve my writing skills. If I was going to finish my dissertation, I had to write what I saw as a short book. Eight years after starting my doctoral studies, I had done very little writing on my dissertation.

Dr. Skovholt, after hearing my story about my wife's threat to divorce me if I didn't finish my doctorate in six months, said he'd meet with me every week and help me write my dissertation. Little did he know, or maybe he did, how much work that helping me complete my writing would entail. In short, he rolled up his sleeves, and helped me form and express my ideas into an acceptable form. I finished my dissertation after six months working with Tom. Needless to say, my development as a writer continues today, as is evident in my being able to sit for hours and days and write this book, which I can share with you takes a lot of technical skill as well as technical writing ability and emotional strength!

I share the latter anecdotes as examples for the importance of having "other support" in order to move to developing "self-support." Fritz Perls, in his book "Gestalt Therapy Verbatim," writes that our development is from "other support to self-support." While Dr. Dolgoff, Dr. Chope, Leroy Gardner, Dr. Skovholt, and so many others, provided me "other support," I needed to develop something else to truly experience my personal growth, namely, learn how to develop true "self-support." However, I didn't know this. I had by 1988 completed my doctoral work, and after teaching psychology courses at California State University, Hayward, I began to work as an administrator at San Francisco State University. But still, I lacked some inner strength to make me more capable of assuming greater responsibility for my life. This would come from my work at the Gestalt Institute of San Francisco; this would come from facing my Childhood Legacy head on!

Becoming Associate Dean of Undergraduate Studies at San Francisco State University was the catalyst that would move me more deeply into Gestalt personal development work. This was a challenge that definitely was another strong "body check" for me. Daily, I would go to work with tense arms and tight legs, and, daily, I would meet the challenge of my work with an unclarified inner resilience, unclarified because I wasn't clear from where my resilience came, nor what it was about.

Let me talk a little about this resilience. First, I say resilience because each day I awoke with tension, and each day I drove to work with tension coursing through my body. I didn't like feeling this way; I didn't like feeling tense and not knowing where this tension came from, nor did I like not knowing what to do about the tension I was experiencing. Take pills? No! Read books? I constantly searched for help regarding body work, such as trying to read Wilhelm Reich's "Character Analysis," or Stanley Keleman's "Your Body Speaks It's Mind," or Sheldon Kopp's "If You Meet the Buddha on the Road, Kill Him" or doing Tai Chi, but I couldn't find within me the passion to continue these avenues of personal development.

My resilience involved my thirst for knowledge about personal growth and the fact that I did not stop searching for an answer to reach my highest form of development, the feeling of freedom and ability to support the daily actions of the person I truly wanted to be! Abraham Maslow, in his book "Toward a Psychology of Being," might offer that within me was the struggle between "the need to know and the fear of knowing" and between "deficiency motivation, maintenance motivation, and actualization motivation." The deficiency motivation I felt was from my Childhood Legacy; the maintenance motivation came from my "fear of knowing;" finally, the "actualization motivation" came from what Perls calls "the need to achieve completeness."

Let me take another non-Gestalt step back. Prior to working at San Francisco State University, I had taught undergraduate courses in psychology at California State University, Hayward, a college that I had attended as an undergraduate in psychology. Significantly, this was a place as a young Latino that I never spoke in class and never raised my hand to ask a question, although it was a place in which I performed well on my exams. I would sometimes go an entire term without speaking in class! The challenge of teaching, especially courses like Abnormal Psychology, where I had to lecture about anxiety disorders, brought me to more and new stress. Again, I had to lecture in courses and classrooms where as an undergraduate I did not speak even once, even though I very much wanted to speak.

A story I share in my talks is that I sometimes had to lecture about panic attacks and the progression of steps during a panic attack, while at the same time I felt like I was having a panic attack! (I vividly recall two young women who every session sat in my class looking at me and giggling about what I thought were impressions of the nervous professor who was in front of them). To meet this challenge, I went back to Dr. Dolgoff and he helped me along my journey by prescribing Ativan, an anti-anxiety medication that reduced my physical tension, thereby allowing me to teach in a calm fashion. After completing my teaching work, I only took Ativan when I had to give talks to large groups, and I continued to take Ativan, although in decreasing amounts over a two-year period, to overcome my fear of speaking in front of large audiences.

Back to San Francisco State University. At one point during my role as Associate Dean of Undergraduate Studies at SFSU, I decided to try further Gestalt work to help me better handle the anxieties that I was daily experiencing in my work and life and the physical stress I was feeling in my body. Because of the beginning work that I had done with Dr. Grossman at the University of Minnesota, I had hope that I could learn to better understand the reason for my anxieties as well as how to "overcome" them. I remembered that during my initial work with Dr. Grossman, I had been able to "stay with my body" through the intense tension that

I experienced in my physical self, especially in my arms and legs. But I recalled it was the competence and skill of Dr. Grossman that gave me the confidence to do difficult Gestalt growth "work." I looked for Gestalt therapists, and I came across an advertisement for the Gestalt Institute of San Francisco. The advertisement talked about "finding yourself," either in individual personal development sessions or in ongoing group sessions. I took a hopeful breath and made an appointment for an individual personal growth session with the director of the institute.

Definitively, without question, my clarity as to my individual identity and potential for development as a unique human being only came about when I turned to the San Francisco Gestalt Institute. Prior to that, I can say that I did not know or have a clear awareness and experience of myself, even though I had read hundreds of personal development and psychology books! The San Francisco Gestalt Institute was for me a combination of individual self-development "work," many months of Friday night three-hour intense group sessions, and unbelievably lively and intense weekend workshops with such Gestalt legends as Dr. Joseph Zinker, Anne Teachworth, Dr. Abe Levitsky, David Schiffman, and Dr. Bud Feeder.

Through these intensely beautiful and memorable experiences (many captured on video), I discovered more and more of my "true self." Increasingly, I became more capable of breathing and releasing tension as I faced challenges to my daily psychological existence. I learned to be more honest and directed with what I felt, thought, and how I wanted to act. I was slowly "leaning into," as Dr. Abe Levitsky would say to us in group meetings, becoming the me I wanted to be!

The person I met when I went to the Gestalt Institute was Morgan Goodlander, a self-styled director who had started Gestalt training when he was sixteen years of age at the Gestalt Institute of New Orleans with an inimitable Gestalt therapist, Anne Teachworth (Anne wrote a fascinating book "Why We Pick the Mates We Do"). Gestalt theory teaches that every action that we take reflects our psychology of being, our stance in life, who we are. Previously, I had read Fritz Perls' book "Gestalt Therapy Verbatim," wherein he wrote about staying with your confusion and trusting your body's natural ability to self-regulate and support the process of personal growth. I definitely had a good deal of confusion in my body and mind, and I hoped that I could sort myself out at the San Francisco Gestalt Institute.

In our first meeting, Morgan listened to me and stared at me intensely, so intensely that I felt that for the first time in my life, someone was really looking at me and watching for what emerged in my physical experience of myself. He watched and listened, and guided me to learn and get in touch with myself, much as I now do with many diverse students and Latin@ community people in my volunteer work in and around Oakland, California. Morgan guided me to do "experiments of growth." Wow! In these "experiments of growth," I learned to trust myself to try new ways of thinking, feeling, and behaving that developed in me more and more the ability to develop "self-support" to be the unique person I am.

Before leaving this chapter, I want to reflect on how my experience of being Latino affected my search for myself in our society. For one, every time I reached out to try and understand myself, especially from a psychological perspective, I did so with a significant feeling of hesitancy and lack of confidence that what I was attempting to do to better myself would help me because I had no one within my family or Latin@ community who served to guide me in my efforts. I think about Dr. Lilia Chavez, a dear colleague and friend of mine whom I introduced to Gestalt. She did a lot of her personal development work from a culturally relevant perspective, and at the same time, I think of myself, who did not have the guidance to do like Lilia. I only had Mario, *Mayito* as my mother and brother called me, to support me to move into a different world of personal psychological study. I think back and realize that much of my efforts were a result of my having "hung around Telegraph Avenue" near UC Berkeley, and catching glimpses during those times of all the various psychological perspectives that existed in the world. Mario moved forward.

Chapter 5

Integrating *FIGURE/GROUND*: Experiments of Growth

In this chapter I share how doing Gestalt personal development work helped me integrate or unify my "self," that is, begin to bring together my past with my present so as to experience and have a more complete self. I share specifics about how the Gestalt personal development work helped me understand how to live in the present and not be controlled by my childhood conditioning, my Childhood Legacy.

I showed up at the Gestalt Institute of San Francisco eager to develop my full potential. Initially, the Institute did not have a home, but rented a meeting space at the San Francisco Integral Counseling Center on the corner of 30th Avenue and Church Street in San Francisco's Noe Valley. The space consisted of two adjoining large rooms, what I imagined were a living room and dining room in a former Victorian home. There were comfortable couches and big pillows spread throughout.

As noted earlier, I was greeted by Morgan Goodlander, a youngish looking man of thirty-something with a big smile, happy eyes, and dark curly hair. I liked his warm-heartedness. We greeted each other, and I shared a little about myself, my background, and what I daily was experiencing related to stress that I wanted to fix, especially the continuous physical tension that I felt in my arms and legs. Over the next three years, I would repeatedly do work with Morgan and other Gestalt therapists that Morgan brought in to conduct Gestalt workshops. What follows are excerpts from key personal development work that I did with Morgan Goodlander and others.

Gestalt Personal Development Sessions
at the Gestalt Institute

First, I will give the sessions a title, and then I will share what occurred in the meeting, and finally, I will share what were for me the important learning aspects of each session. At the end of this chapter, I will summarize my overall learning experiences gained in my personal development work at the Gestalt Institute, and, especially, how each session allowed for more and more integration (unification) of my unique experience as Mario Rivas.

The Cartoon/Angry Dog/
Vulnerable Little Latino Boy Sessions

Morgan: Tell me what you feel in your arms.

Mario: I feel tension in my arms, but there's no direction for the tension, like there's something I want to do, but I don't know what it is!

Morgan: Stay with the feeling.

Morgan watched every part of me for how I/my body reacted to his request to stay with my feelings. The intensity of his gaze was at the same time disarming and somewhat comical. Disarming, because I saw someone really focused on my growth, and comical in that Morgan was not guarding his facial or physical expressions, so sometimes I would see what I considered a funny face or funny bodily postures. Initially I was distracted, but soon I went back into my personal work, accepting the honesty and caring nature of Morgan's attentive interaction with me.

Morgan: I see that you take a big breath when I ask you to focus on the tension in your arms. Can you repeat that?

Take another deep breath.

I did so, and I "found" myself and "experienced" myself becoming more energized. Wow! Where was this going? I felt my eyes beginning to water (an experience that I would repeat over and over again in the next three years of doing Gestalt "work," so much so that Dr. Joseph Zinker, a Gestalt genius (to me and so many others), would say that he had never met a person who so quickly could go into deep emotions, especially those related to hurt and fear. Morgan did not miss my eyes welling up with tears again, much as I now don't miss tears welling up in students as I do Gestalt work with them at conferences or groups that I have worked with at Merritt College, San Francisco State University, Berkeley City College, and in the Oakland-East Bay Latin@ community.

Morgan: What are you experiencing?

Mario: I don't know. I feel like I want to cry.

Morgan: Stay with that feeling. Stay with yourself, your experience.

The tears came. I cried and cried and cried. Where was I going? What did these tears mean? Whew! This experience of myself was really intense!

Morgan: Close your eyes.

I acceded.

Morgan: What do you see? What do you feel?

Mario: Wow! I see a jumbled mess of colors, incomplete fragments of actions, exclamation marks, number signs, all mixed together like one sees in cartoons where the characters are entangled in a chaotic battle, fight.

Morgan: Stay with this image. What do you feel?

Mario: The image is overwhelming. It goes nowhere, nothing forms. Nothing becomes clear, just this mixed bag of negative, intense energy jumbled onto and within itself.

There are no distinct feelings, just this overwhelming picture of chaos.

I "stayed" with this image. (I have, over the years, come to understand this image as my initial experience of my undiscovered, lost, incomplete self that had started to form in childhood, and was thrown into chaos in great part because of my confused and abusive father. I now imagine that in my adulthood, I was mixed up within my emotions and bodily sensations, the ones that I had accumulated during my Childhood Legacy. But more of this later.)

Morgan: What do you feel toward this image?

Mario: I feel it's foreign. I feel like I'm on the outside, only a witness to what's going on. No, not even a witness, more an observer who doesn't have any idea about what he's seeing. My feeling: feelings of being lost, confused, mixed up. I am not in touch with the picture!

Morgan: Put the picture on one of these pillows. Do you want to say anything to the picture?

A big part of Gestalt work is to learn to become aware of how we physically experience our self. One way of doing this is by looking at different aspects of our self by externalizing the experience. In this latter piece of work, Morgan asked me to place the chaotic cartoon-like image on a pillow. He then supported me to interact with the image so that I could get a feel for and understanding of this experience.

Mario: (Interacting with the cartoon-like picture): I don't understand you; I don't know what you're about, what you want to communicate to me.

Morgan: (Watching me intently) What does your body say to you as you look at this picture?

Mario: I have no sensation, no energy. I feel like I cannot move.

I would revisit and see this scene over and over in my future Gestalt work with Morgan and others, and eventually a FIGURE would form out of the unclarified GROUND that was my experience of my early life, especially my Childhood Legacy. The figure that would eventually form from this jumbled confusion of strong unbridled energy was my experience of myself, although seeing an image of me was not what I initially saw. In fact, the first clear perceptions I had of the picture were initially a fierce set of teeth, and then I eventually reached out and fearfully touched a hard, very rough surface.

I could almost taste the action of touching the hard surface — a bitter, harsh taste. This was a taste that made me want to spit out with abhorrence and rejection. In time and after more work, I saw a fuzzy tanned surface that was also scary for me to touch. But ever so slowly in my imagination, touch I did. Eventually, I saw horrifying, growling teeth and then the face of a huge, angry dog, something like a mastiff. In retrospect, this image must have been some image that I conjured up from one of those angry cartoon scenarios I watched as a little boy.

Behind this angry dog, I was eventually able to see my little boy self, who in my Gestalt work, over time, would move slowly from a fearful and then angry, rejecting child to a little boy who gradually accepted my efforts to connect to him with love and caring. I would learn more and more of my confusion of pent-up feelings — of my fear, anger, hurt, rage, feeling of being lost, etc. I feel teary at this moment, recalling this unformed FIGURE, what I will call an undifferentiated mass of emotions whose only image was represented by what I had seen in cartoon fights.

In my Gestalt personal development work, I have

learned that my tears, my emotional reaction to my vulnerable little boy self, signal to me that I still need to do more work with this image, this unfinished, incomplete gestalt. I'm excited by the possibility of becoming more aware and clearer about who I am at the present because of the legacy of my past, especially of the time when I was a vulnerable little Costa Rican kid in the U.S.A.

I was hooked on Gestalt personal development work. I always left Morgan's office with hope that this work that I did with him would lead me to a greater wholeness, completeness, and greater ability to be and express myself directly, honestly, and assertively with others. I remembered Fritz Perls' statement in his book "Gestalt Therapy Verbatim," where he asserts, "It is our birthright to achieve completeness." I thought, 'Is this possible? Can I really complete myself? And what does that even mean?'"

At this point, I had earned a bachelor's degree in psychology, a master's degree in counseling, and a Ph.D. in counseling and student personnel psychology, but I felt only about 70 percent complete within myself — 70 percent being a general figure that said to me that I had come a long way in my personal development, but needed to keep going to continue experiencing more growth and feelings of personal empowerment in my ability to think, feel, and act consistent with my values and beliefs. Was more completeness possible, especially since I didn't definitively know what being complete meant? I hoped, yes! For years to come, I would continue with my Gestalt personal development work in search of more completeness, including having a greater understanding and experience of what individual completeness means. Let me continue sharing my personal growth journey through the use of Gestalt personal development work.

The Witch-Broom/Scared Little Boy Session

Another significant piece of work related to my personal development, my search for completeness, came during the time that I taught my first undergraduate course at San Francisco State University in 1996. I had previously taught graduate courses at SFSU in counseling, including multicultural counseling, college counseling, and undergraduate courses in psychology at CSU Hayward including social psychology, and abnormal psychology, but now my uniqueness was being tested because I had to teach a "mandatory" course on how to face the challenges of college that would be required of all freshman students at SFSU, many of whom would turn out to be unwilling enrollees in the course, and who would question, often in an angry way, why they had to take such a course.

This course was the idea of the SFSU Mandatory Advising Task Force, which was charged to increase student persistence and success at the university. I was assigned to be chair of this group, and, yes, I again was filled with fear. (Have I made a clear point that I just didn't walk into being successful as a professional with ease, grace, and unbridled confidence?) This 'little Latino welfare street kid from North Oakland, California,' as I often saw myself, was now in charge of a committee of powerful faculty members at San Francisco State University, and as committee chair, I was charged to develop a mandatory advising policy and related interventions that would make a difference in students' persistence and success at the university.

Again, one of the major recommendations of this task force was that a course be developed to help freshmen students more effectively start their studies at the university.

With the help of colleagues such as Dr. Gerald Eisman, Department Chair of Computer Science, Dr. Phil McGee, Dean of the College of Ethnic Studies, Dr. Susan Taylor, Dean of the College of Behavioral and Social Sciences, Dr. Nancy Mc Dermitt, Dean of the College of Humanities, Dr. Susan Schiminoff, Department Chair of Speech and Communications, and other highly competent faculty and administrators, we developed and prepared to offer a mandatory freshman orientation course during the fall of 1998. And, I was chosen as the first instructor! Not too much pressure, huh?

Being only mildly confident about teaching the freshman course, I started to experience a considerable amount of anxiety, and my anxiety became increasingly more intense when a group of about twenty of the one-hundred-plus enrolled students started to balk and react negatively about being in the class. Every class meeting, this group of students sat at the back and communicated their displeasure at having to be in the class, and they showered me with looks of dislike and disinterest. My anxiety became stronger and stronger every time I thought about teaching the class, and increased as I approached each class session. I can feel some of the stress in my shoulders and calves and the tightness in my chest at this present moment as I remember the tense feelings I experienced when thinking about or when teaching the class.

I stop now and stay with my feelings and I can see an image as I experience these feelings in the present. This image is a mixture of my scared little boy and the ferocious, angry dog I have previously mentioned, but also of the adult professor standing in front of the class. I experiment, and imagine holding my little boy self in my arms, even though he's a somewhat frightening expression of anger and rage.

I hold him and assure him I love him, and at the same time, I breathe deeply and assure myself that my experience of me is a truthful acting out of self-support.

I stay with the present tension in my shoulders and forearms, a different tension than in the past — a more self-assured, deliberate and intentional tension that is focused on writing this book. I breathe deeply, almost automatically now because of the extensive Gestalt work that I've done to free myself of my Childhood Legacy, of being a vulnerable and incapable little boy. My angry, rage-filled little boy recedes more into the background, and a new mental figure forms of a little boy holding my hand and walking with me down a tree-lined path, although the angry little boy breaks through from time to time.

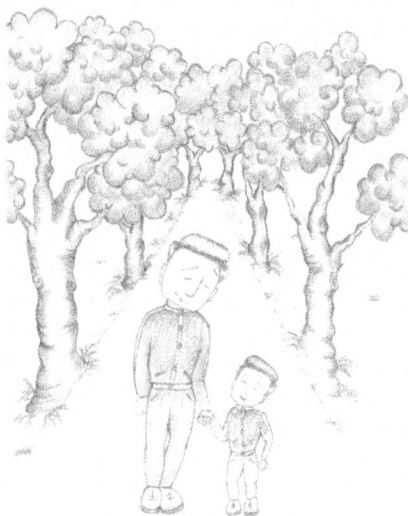

In my imagination, the ferocious dog is to the side watching carefully what is transpiring between the little boy and me. I smile and relax more. I'll go back and do more work

with this image in the future, again, work that is called "unfinished business" by Gestalt therapists. But now, back to
the group of resentful students at SFSU who were challenging my unique expression of self, me in the process of developing my completeness as Mario. I called Morgan at the
Gestalt Institute, my "other-support" in my progression to
"self-support," and made an appointment to do work with
the anxiety I was experiencing.

As I would experience many times in the future, I
showed up to Morgan with hope that I could do work to
meet this anxiety-filled growth challenge of mine. I shared
with Morgan what I was experiencing in the class, the anxiety and doubt, and then he asked me the following question.

Morgan: Tell me what you experience when you see an
image of the resentful students?

Mario: Well, I feel a mixture of anger and resentment
from them, and I want this group of students to stop being
angry at me and accept me.

Morgan looked intently at me and studied me.

Morgan: Why don't you try an experiment with me, and
imagine your little boy sitting among these students.

Mario: Okay.

Morgan: What do you see?

Mario: Well, I see my little boy, and . . .

Morgan: Yes, what do you see?

Mario: I don't know. There's something above the little
boy which is hard for me to make out.

Morgan: Stay with the image. What do you see?

Mario: Well, it looks like a witch with a broom. Wow,
that's weird!

I feel a twinge of dizziness in the present as I recall this image. This is another example of "unfinished business," because my mind through my body is signaling to me that I have leftover feelings of doubt, fear, and anxiety that I have learned, which stem in great part from my Childhood Legacy.

Morgan: Why don't we do some chair work with that witch with the broom?

What is Gestalt Chair Work?

I want to discuss a little more about Gestalt chair work. Fritz Perls did chair work as a way to help persons experience, get in touch with, and integrate a split in the self that persons often develop as they experience life challenges, when self-acceptance and self-support are undermined. Again, this occurs especially during childhood when we are more psychologically vulnerable to negative experiences. For example, for me, I have shared that the personal childhood experiences created a "little Mario who felt lost, hurt, confused, etc." Such experiences often create a split in a person where one part of the self is preferred, and the other, usually more weak and doubtful part of the self is rejected.

(I keep thinking that "completeness" may have to do when we accept all parts of ourselves. Also, completeness may not be a state we achieve once and for all; rather, it may be a process wherein we daily accept ourselves more and more and listen and rely on all parts of our self-experience as we face life's psychological challenges. I will come back to this later).

Fritz Perls called the often-conflicting aspects of our self-strong and weak- the "top dog and underdog," respectively. The "top dog" is that part of ourselves that often chides, criticizes, judges, looks down on, prods, and directs us to be strong and meet challenges head-on, e.g., 'You're stupid, weak, not likeable.' The underdog is that part of the self which is often experienced as vulnerable, weak, fearful, undirected, less confident, and less capable of handling challenges, e.g., 'I'll never be able to, I really am weak, I don't deserve...' (This reminds me of my vulnerable little boy). The chair work pits these two polar opposites (called polarities in Gestalt personal development work because there often exist polar opposites within the personality) against one another, which under the skillful support of a Gestalt therapist, leads to a resolution and integration of the split wherein following the work the individual experiences an awareness of self as more united, integrated, and complete (see Fritz Perls' book "Gestalt Therapy Verbatim" for a good explanation and examples of this chair work).

In chair work, usually consisting of two chairs (but there can be more chairs), the person doing the work switches back and forth, assuming each position, again, either as the "top dog or underdog." In short, I see the power of this method to be that the person doing the work directly experiences aspects of his/her-self that have heretofore not been totally and separately experienced, and that are often split off from the person's sense of self or developing completeness. This experiencing of different aspects of self builds a more complete body-mind integration of all possible alternatives when facing daily life challenges.

Back to Morgan's work with me experiencing my little boy in the midst of the angry and resentful students with the witch with a broom standing over little Mario.

Morgan: Sit in the chair here and be the little boy. What do you experience as that little boy? What do you feel?

Mario: Well, the little boy is afraid. He's afraid that the witch is going to hurt him. He wants to hide. His head wants to turn away, and he feels like cowering in the corner (this I see as the "underdog").

Morgan: Don't talk about Little Mario. Be him.

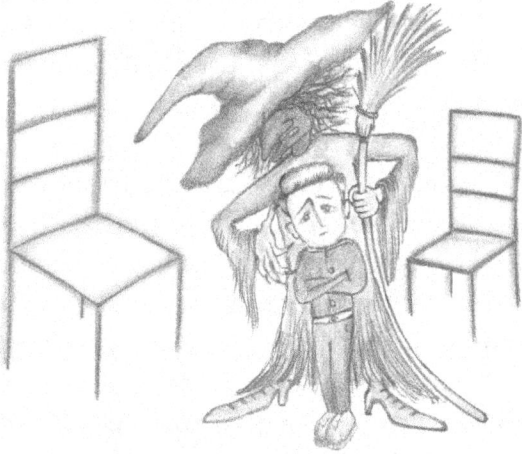

Little Mario: I am afraid. I want to run away and hide! (In Spanish, *Yo quiero alejarme y esconderme!*)

Morgan: I notice your chest being energized more and more, and your lips are trembling. Does Little Mario want to say something to the witch?

Mario: Yes.

Morgan: Go ahead. Speak to the witch from the energy that you feel in your chest, in your trembling lips.

Little Mario: A welling up of energy in the little boy's chest, and he blurts out: No! (The no is a Spanish-accented no!)

Morgan: Change chairs and be the witch. What is her reaction? Does she say anything?

Mario as the witch: The witch is feeling strong anger

and resentment toward the little boy, and a powerful, potent strength in her arms: *Cayate, chiquillo malo! Le voy a decir a su papa!* (Shut up, you bad boy. I'm going to tell your father!).

(I see the witch as the "top dog," that part of Mario who judges himself as wrong, bad, not capable, not worthy of love, and who wants Mario to be a copy of what she thinks he should be. The way the top dog in me thinks I should be with the students: tough, strong, confident, controlling, taking charge.)

Morgan then asked me if I could recognize the witch lady, and I said I couldn't. He asked me to speak to my mother and brother about this witch, and ask them if she represented anybody they knew. The session ended.

That night, I visited my mama who was in the hospital, and I asked her if she or "mamita" (my grandmother in Costa Rica whom I knew when I lived there as a little boy) or anyone else who had been mean to me when I was little. My mother emphatically said no; she did not recall any such person. I explained to mama the work I was doing, and how I was trying to learn how my childhood affected my ability to be a confident man at work and in my life. I shared with her that this witch was possibly a representation of some person or experience in my childhood that had a powerful effect on my ability to face situations where people are angry with me. My beautiful mama paid attention to me and seemed to drift into deep thought. *"Tal vez fue en Costa Rica cuando tubiste que ir a la casa de Rosa, su tia, la hermana de su papa. Cuando volviste estabas lleno de miedo y terror y lloraste que nunca querias volver alli. Y nunca volviste!"* The following is a translation of what my mother shared with me.

"Maybe it was your aunt Rosa, your father's sister. When you returned from visiting her one time, you were extremely afraid and filled with terror and you cried that you never wanted to return there, and you never did!" Wow! Maybe the witch was an image related to the negative emotions that I had internalized from my experience with my aunt Rosa, whom I only saw once in my life, because I was so afraid of her that I refused to see her again. The key point here is that my childhood experience, whether real or imagined, resulted in my internalizing a legacy of fear related to me being a fearful child in the face of a challenging situation.

Amazingly, when I returned to my next class meeting, my anxiety was much less, and I was able to walk with a positive energy to the back of the classroom and address the concerns of the students more directly. How did this happen? From a Gestalt perspective, I can say that I carried in my body and deep sensory memory the unfinished business of the fear and terror of having to face what I perceived as my angry aunt, who I felt didn't accept me, and that this was projected onto the students in my class at SFSU. Also, a major benefit of my chair work is that I physically reexperienced my child self, thereby redoing my physically and psychologically internalized fears. I directly faced part of my Childhood Legacy, and reexperienced my imaginary "angry witch." This freed me from my early "emotional binds" (What Perls referred to as emotional barriers to personal integration and growth) to be able to experiment with some new behavior with the students in the present. At a deeper level, I interpret the polarity I carried within myself as the "top dog in me," learned from my experience with my tough father and aunt, pushing me to be tough and angry and strong with the students, while the "underdog" or scared part of me wanted to run away and hide.

I have come to "understand" my experience in the class-room as a somatic (body), emotional reaction to a strong subconscious memory that was associated with a person being angry with me. Also, I have come to understand that if I face these same emotions in the present with trust in my ability to "stay with the emotions and not run away," I can learn how to use the psychological resources of my adult self to support me to re-do and finish a previously unfin-ished and not understood challenging emotional experience.

The Angry Vice President/Father/Fearful Associate Dean/Little Boy "Dizzy" Session

The next experience of Gestalt growth work also relates to an experience I had while working as Associate Dean of Undergraduate Studies at San Francisco State University. This situation involved an instance where I had been charged to oversee a new academic program that reported directly to the California State University Chancellor's Of-fice. As part of this responsibility, I had hurriedly hired a program director, and we were one month into the program. Both the program director and I were "newbies" to the pro-gram. Nonetheless, a month into the program, we were charged to write a year-end program report. I remember whipping up a report with the director as best as we could.

Alarmingly, I was called into the Office of the Vice Pres-ident of Instruction, whom I perceived to be stern man and who inspired caution, doubt, and fear in me. The Vice Pres-ident demanded that I give an account of why the report was so incomplete! I remember standing in front of the Vice President as he spoke in a stern voice.

"This report is unacceptable! It is written poorly and isn't well organized. What do you have to say for yourself?" he asked.

"Well," I answered. "We've only had the program one month, and I and the program director did the best we could."

"Is that it? Is that all you can offer me?" replied the Vice President.

"Yes," I said, but I was upset and fearful, and couldn't express more.

The Vice President finished with, "Your response and this work is unacceptable!"

I left his office shaking with emotion. I was angry that I had been treated with what I perceived as shabbily disrespectful by the Vice President, and I was upset with myself that I had not stood up and expressed myself in a more effective, assertive manner. At the same time, I was fearful of what this would mean to my job. I made an appointment with Morgan at the Gestalt Institute.

I notice that I often say that I turned to Morgan for help with my anxiety, and I want to briefly address how I see the need to have more therapists and counselors available to the general public, especially Latin@ and other diverse ethnic counselors. I was fortunate to have reached a stage in my life when I could afford reaching out for help, and I was fortunate to have been able to search for the right help; however, I know too many people who are not afforded this experience or opportunity. Indeed, this should be a right that we all have in such an advanced and wealthy society! This again is one reason that I am writing this book, because, generally, individuals from diverse ethnic backgrounds, and especially, persons with little money, do not have the luxury to call and make an appointment with a psychologist or counselor. We need more of this support for the persons who have too little social and economic capital, and I hope this book helps persons, community agencies, and government programs to develop centers of personal growth (e.g., mini-Gestalt-like institutes) where more and more people can be helped to face their psychological challenges.

In the meeting with Morgan, I shared my experience with the Vice President of Instruction, and Morgan quickly had me do some chair work, where I was in one chair and the Vice President was in the other chair.

Mario as Vice President: "This work is unacceptable!"

Morgan advised me to really get into the role of the Vice President, and deeply experience his emotions and persona (personality characteristics).

Morgan: What do you feel?

Mario: I feel strong. I feel like I belong, like I'm the boss. I feel like I can make things happen!

Morgan: Where do you feel this in your body?

Mario: All over my body, but especially in my chest and arms.

Morgan: Stand up and repeat, as Vice President, your statement to Mario.

I did so, and responded to Morgan's question of my experience that I felt strong and powerful. Morgan went on.

Morgan: Now sit in the chair as Mario, the Associate Dean of Undergraduate Studies.

I did so.

Morgan: What do you experience, feel?

Mario: I feel weak. I feel like I don't belong. I experience myself as wanting to be strong, but I don't know how to do that. My chest feels deflated; my shoulders drop; my arms are tense and nervous.

Morgan: What do you want to say to the Vice President? What do you need from him?

Mario: I want to say that he is being unfair, that he needs to be more understanding and supportive.

Morgan: Go ahead.

Mario as Associate Dean: I think you're being unfair, unjust. I did not have much experience with this program, and I did the best I could. Also, I think that you are not acknowledging how valuable I am here at SFSU as well as supporting me to develop in this role!

Morgan: How do you feel? What is your experience?

Mario: I don't feel much, because I experience myself as only asking for something and not getting it. I feel incomplete (I feel that this feeling of getting what one wants is part of what achieving completeness means).

Morgan: Let's try an experiment. Sit in the Vice President's chair and be what you perceive would be a good, caring, and supportive Vice President. Give Mario what he wants and needs. Recognize his importance to SFSU; recognize how special he is. Tell him how you want to support his development.

I got up from the Mario chair and went to go to the VP's chair. Immediately I became dizzy, so much so that I almost fell over. This feeling was strange and scary, but under the caring gaze of Morgan, I balanced myself, and moved tentatively to the VP's chair. (I feel a twinge of dizziness in my head right now as I write, and at the same time and almost automatically, I take a big breath that balances me. I know that this sequence of doubt and fear, coupled with a breath of strength and resolve, reflects my psychologically developing self, which results from my repeated Gestalt work).

Morgan encouraged me to continue with the exercise. I took a stabilizing breath and sat in the VP's chair to be a "good, caring, supportive VPI."

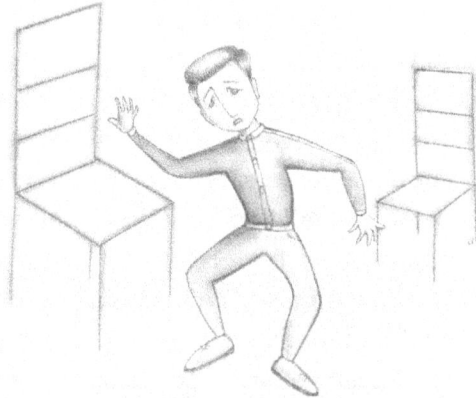

Good, caring, supportive VPI: Mario, I want you to know that this report could have been done much, much better, and to that end, I want to meet with you and the new director and work with you to prepare a better report next time. Also, I want you to know that I and so many others in this university value you a lot; we see your importance and care for you so much! Also, I want you to know that as a leader here I value your work, and I support you 100 percent. I want you to trust yourself, your creativity, and your strength, to do good things on behalf of students, and I want you to feel free to come and talk to me anytime you want about any ideas, concerns or needs you have, and I want you to know that I'm always available to support and work with you!

Wow! In that moment, I broke into tears and couldn't stop crying, which I did for a good amount of time. (I feel teary-eyed now remembering this work, and I realize how valuable "other support" is for our growth. I also realize that chair work helps one internalize and integrate emotions that in our life were part of incomplete experiences/gestalts, experiences where we rejected within ourselves difficult emotions, holding and not integrating [making part of us] emotions that if internalized in a positive and complete manner we could rely on to face difficult personal development emergencies, e.g., needing to feel care and support toward one's self when needed.)

Morgan patiently let me experience myself completely. I become teary-eyed reflecting on that statement: "Morgan let me experience myself completely." (Does achieving completeness involve repeated situations wherein a person 'stays with their experience of "self," becoming more and more familiar with the experience of feeling complete as a person who thinks, feels and behaves in a unique way? And does completeness involve becoming more and more aware of the process of completing life situations that are challenging? Very, very interesting.)

I felt drained after the Associate Dean/VPI Gestalt work, and I think I learned and experienced something very important. I experienced what is called a "complete gestalt" where I was valued (I think this relates to Laura Rendon's Validation Theory, wherein she argues that many Latin@s and people of color don't experience much validation in our society, and, therefore, we need this experience from professors and other professionals to psychologically support our efforts to succeed in college and career). In this experience and in many that would follow, I learned that I had many "incomplete gestalts" that came from my Childhood Legacy.

One major incomplete gestalt (unfinished business) is

that I never had the "other support" of a loving, accepting, supportive father, when I could build, breathe into my body, a complete gestalt wherein I could stand as a unique person and feel strength, self-support, and self-acceptance. I was now learning to do this in my present Gestalt work by being, embodying, the loving and caring VPI. I was transforming an internalized negative non-supportive father and, instead, integrating within my mind and body a powerful, caring, and loving father/authority figure who through the chair work experience I was becoming! Wow! This Gestalt work was really making a difference in my life!

The "What Does Your Hurt Little Boy Need?" Session

The next anecdote I want to share has to do with an example of Gestalt work that helped me further clarify how my Childhood Legacy was affecting me in the present, both in my personal and professional life. Before sharing the story, I want to reemphasize the phrase that I came up with to explain the importance of doing Gestalt work so as to learn how not to have one's present be overly influenced by negative emotional learning experiences from one's past. Again, the phrase is the following: "Our future will be our past, unless we bring our past into our present, and choose our future!"

By this saying, I want to re-emphasize that Gestalt personal development work involves more than just "talking about" the difficulties and challenges that all of us bring to the present from our past. Gestalt work involves actually re-experiencing the past by bringing the past, including learned and internalized emotions and behaviors, into the present in the same form, but experimenting with changing and developing new responses to past traumas. These new responses allow for individuals to choose more effective ways of being in the present and future, ways that let go of the past and use the capabilities and personal strengths of the adult self to support acting in self-affirming, self-supportive, and self-directing ways.

Later, I will share how through Gestalt Educational Counseling (GEC), a brand of Gestalt counseling that I developed, I teach persons, especially persons like myself, a first-generation Latino in the U.S.A., to become educated about how to use psychology, and Gestalt personal development work in particular, to improve the ability to handle life's psychological challenges.

In my "What does your hurt little boy need?" piece of Gestalt work, I was introduced more completely to my little boy, and especially how my Childhood Legacy was so much a part of how I was facing my adult life. While working as Associate Dean of Undergraduate Studies at San Francisco State University, I gave numerous keynote addresses at professional conferences as well as to faculty, administrators, and staff at many colleges and universities around the nation, and also to many student groups. As you may recall, my initial experience of lecturing in classes as well as giving speeches produced much anxiety in me.

Also, you'll recall that Dr. Robert Dolgoff prescribed Ativan, a benzodiazepine that "makes nerves less sensitive to stimulation." This medication calmed my overactive sympathetic nervous system to help me relax the anxiety I experienced when having to speak in front of groups. The pill worked, but I did not think that by taking a pill to handle my life's challenges I was directing and truly taking charge of my life. Rather, I felt that I was using pills as a crutch that allowed me to be only a part of myself. I didn't feel good with that, and even though I shared my use of Ativan to audiences when I made presentations, I still felt that I was not being true to the person I wanted to be — independent, autonomous, self-directed, self-supporting — all the good stuff I've come to know that all of us want to be!

In my now regular meetings with Morgan Goodlander, the Director of the Gestalt Institute of San Francisco, I brought up that while I stopped using Ativan when I lectured in the classroom, I nevertheless was taking half of a milligram tablet (a small dosage) when I gave speeches in front of large groups. Such a talk was coming up where I was to present to the entire faculty at Dominican University in San Rafael, California. I was feeling anxious as the day of the talk approached and I told Morgan that I was thinking about taking the half milligram tablet of Ativan, but that I did not feel good about doing that. Morgan asked me to not take the tablet and, instead, on the way to the talk, to ask my "little boy" what he needed. As a lead up to this, Morgan asked me to draw simple pictures of my little boy crying and place them around my house, and, when seeing the picture, to ask my crying, hurt little boy what he needed. I did this.

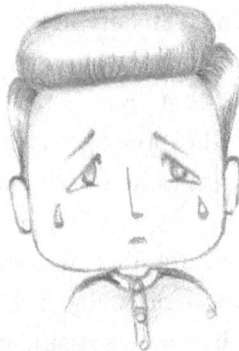

Doing this exercise helped me get in touch with how much I had never known or been truly aware of my childhood pain. The little boy's crying face evoked feelings in me of hurt, sadness, and compassion. Whenever I looked at the face and asked the little boy what he needed, I inevitably got responses like the following: I need for you to love me; I need for you to take care of me; I need for you to understand me; I need for you to be strong . . . Whew! This, in the language of me as a little boy wanting to be supported and loved.

On the drive to Dominican College after not taking Ativan, I asked my little boy what he needed, and I had to pull over because I again began to cry deeply and intensely. I did get to my talk, and I gave what I thought was an inspiring presentation, but this time, without taking Ativan! I felt I was becoming more of me, freeing myself from the fears and doubts of my past. And, since that time, some twenty-five years ago, I have not taken Ativan again!

For me, I understood that now I was truly in touch with my "little boy," and I could do work with him directly as I needed, rather than bypassing awareness of the present-day effects of my childhood hurts with the use of medication. Looking back, I also think that if I had turned to Gestalt personal development work before Dr. Dolgoff, I may never have taken any medication to help me "be me." In fact, I know this for a fact, because I have seen hundreds of cases where doing Gestalt work has either freed persons from taking medication or stopped the need to do so.

I am reminded of an occasion when I did personal work that involved imagining and working directly with my little boy. One was after my divorce when I was in a relationship with a young woman whom I loved very much. Our relationship had lasted for nearly five years. At one point, she broke off our relationship to be with a younger man. I was devastated. I remember that I felt lost without her, so much so, that I would drive by her house in hope of not seeing the other young man's car. I did this against my will, because I thought in my mind that this behavior wasn't good for me developing my inner strength to handle difficult interpersonal challenges.

Nevertheless, I did this behavior because I did not know what else to do to relieve my pain of being alone and separated from a person so special to me. One Friday night after the weekly three-hour Gestalt group at the now physically real Gestalt Institute on 330 Balboa Street in San Francisco, I felt impelled to drive by the house of my former girlfriend. In the group, I shared this behavior, and Morgan suggested that rather than driving by the house, I instead park and ask my little boy what he needed.

I did this, and I again did my usual intense crying, but then an image of my hurt little boy emerged when I was at St. Vincent's School for Boys, seemingly alone without my mama. To my question of what he needed, my little-boy-self answered that he needed for me to love him, be with him, and support him in his feeling of aloneness and feeling lost. Wow, as I reread this, I feel a sense of goodness in my body that I think comes with my learning to support myself to stay with, hold, and grow through difficult internalized feelings that I had experienced in childhood when I did not have the psychological strength to handle difficult emotions.

I recall that sitting in my car I told myself that I would experiment with this new way of handling my personal pain of losing contact with a loved one, and I immediately drove home without doing a "drive-by" to my former girlfriend's house! Also, I never repeated this behavior, ever, and instead when I had feelings of hurt, I did Gestalt work with my little-boy-self to progressively reintegrate my childhood negative feelings with the strength of my present, more resilient, and psychologically developed self.

Ever since working with my" "little-boy-self," I have more and more been able to support myself to be steady and present with my experience of self, even though at times continuing to experience feelings of doubt, fear, hopelessness, insecurity, etc. Through persistent Gestalt work, I have progressively integrated my Childhood Legacy of doubt, fear, hopelessness, confusion, etc. into my adult being, but this time with more "self-support." As Fritz Perls might say, I have matured, and am now more capable of directing myself, expressing myself, and being more assertive and responsible to face the normal psychological challenges that one faces in everyday life.

One area in my life where I have made use of Gestalt personal development concepts is in my professional work as a counseling psychologist, both in my teaching and Gestalt work supporting students to develop their strength to be successful in college, as well as in my volunteer community work, either helping persons improve their ability to negotiate the challenges of life, or in mentoring persons of color and others to learn to use Gestalt for themselves and to help others develop psychological strength. I now turn to this.

Chapter 6

Professional Growth:
I Develop Gestalt Educational Counseling (GEC)

I've shared how Gestalt personal development work helped me face personal and professional challenges related to managing my emotions and developing a more effective and complete personality. I've shared that I achieved a greater completeness in my personality because of the awareness I developed regarding the mistaken and negative beliefs that I developed because of my Childhood Legacy. I've also shared that I became aware of how my Childhood Legacy was internalized in my body in the nervousness I felt in my arms and legs and the dizziness I felt in my brain, especially when I faced personal and professional challenges. I've also shared that my life's work is to help others who are in need of psychological support. I now want to pass on how I developed my unique approach to using Gestalt personal development methods to help college students face emotional challenges, and especially Latin@s and other students of color to develop greater strength to manage emotional and psychological challenges in their studies and life in general.

This section chronicles how I have continued to develop as a person and professional. As a person, because I have continued on a unique path for how I want to complete myself and as a professional because I have continued to focus my professional efforts, even into retirement, to using what I call Gestalt Educational Counseling to support the psychological growth of individuals and community groups, especially Latin@ and people of color.

My Motivation and Early Experiences in
Developing Gestalt Educational Counseling (GEC)

At this point, I want to share thoughts and experiences related to the development of my professional self, especially as it relates to my identity as a Latino in the U.S.A., and how I developed GEC. First, my Latino identity has always been at work in my career development. A favorite quote of my good friend and colleague Tom Brown is that a career is something you do for yourself, and a job is something you do for somebody else. In this regard, my career has been a continual progression to become and express my unique self. I didn't just complete a generic master's and doctoral degree and follow a predictable career path. No, I have lived out a "career self" who has stayed true to holding on to values and beliefs that reflect an integration of my Latin@ culture in the U.S.A. and the social experience within my family of origin.

In this process, I have constantly searched for satisfaction and passion in what I do as a career. In my career, I have constantly searched for how I can share with others what I consider to be essential to what it means to complete oneself as a person. Gestalt personal development concepts have supported both my personal and professional development because the principles of Gestalt therapy exemplify the freedom of being congruent/consistent with and expressing one's true self. In my career development, I stayed true to helping others, a central value of Latin@ culture.

Why did I develop my own brand of using Gestalt work with students and community groups? There are two reasons. As you will recall, my Latina mama instilled in me the value of helping less fortunate people to have fulfilling lives:

"Lo mas importante en la vida es ayudar a nuestro proximo!" In
Oakland, California, the community of my childhood where
there were many diverse persons, this mantra of my mama
influenced me as a professional to want to be of service to
lower income people, especially people of color, to support
ourselves to become more knowledgeable psychologically
so as to live more complete, satisfying, and fulfilling lives.

With respect to my own Chicano/Latino community, my
mama's value instilled in me a drive to help my community
— *"mi gente."* I went to the University of Minnesota to do
doctoral work in counseling psychology with this intent,
and, subsequently, my professional work has always been
colored by my mama's values and my social experiences as
a Latino in Oakland and the surrounding San Francisco Bay
Area. A sad and chilling experience related to my wanting
to focus my doctoral study on helping Latin@ community
members is a statement made to me by a Anglo faculty
member in my doctoral program during my first month at
the University of Minnesota. I can see us stepping off a curb
on the tree-lined street in front of Burton Hall on the University of Minnesota campus and being asked, "Can't you
Latinos focus on something other than helping your community?" This shocked me at that moment, and made me
question whether my graduate study focus was an appropriate area to do research and practice. I can imagine that if
this prestigious faculty member would have helped me define my intentions more clearly as well as clarify how to research my personal vision, my doctoral studies would have
been more directly related to my initial values and vision.
But this was not so.

While my lack of initial support from some of my graduate faculty led me to change my focus from strictly

studying how to empower Latino families and individuals to master our nation's educational system, I did not give up on helping underprepared students of color, those having backgrounds similar to mine, to become more empowered and effective in their pursuit of success in higher education. Ironically, I recently participated on a doctoral committee for a Latina whose main goal is to help Latinos and families of color to better navigate higher education!

By way of background for how I arrived at the use of Gestalt counseling methods, I want to digress to my early work as a counselor before I learned to understand and use Gestalt principles and practices of personal growth. In my beginning work as a counselor at Valley College in Livermore, California between 1976 and 1979, I emphasized interpersonal openness as a way of becoming more self-secure as a person. I taught classes on improving self-esteem and interpersonal communication, using books like Joseph Powell's "Why am I Afraid to Tell You Who I Am?" William Schutz' book "Joy," Nathaniel Branden's "The Psychology of Self-Esteem," and Erich Fromm's "The Art of Loving."

I found that supporting persons to be more open and trusting toward themselves and others was a good way to help them to develop psychological strength and confidence. What I did not know was that there was an even more powerful way of helping myself and others take control of our lives than merely opening up to self and others about strengths and vulnerabilities. Still, there was a kernel of truth in the mantra of interpersonal openness that is congruent with Gestalt personal development work, which is to stay with yourself and be true to what you feel is your personal essence regarding how to live life.

In my professional work as a college educator, my

increasing knowledge of Gestalt theory and practice led me to want to give the power and benefits of Gestalt personal development work to students. Therefore, as Associate Dean of Undergraduate Studies at San Francisco State University, I initially volunteered my time to work with Latin@ students at the La Raza Student Organization. I recall with pride and fondness how this group of students opened themselves up and allowed me to teach and introduce them to Gestalt work through use of the technique called "La Silla Vacia" (The Empty Chair Technique). I worked with these students in bimonthly group sessions. My interest in making Gestalt more available to less affluent populations was buoyed by the genuine acceptance on the part of La Raza Student Organization at SFSU, and this interest continued in my next position at Vista Community College in Berkeley, California.

My next career position was as Vice President of Student Services at Vista Community College, now Berkeley City College. Part of my personal challenge was how I could use Gestalt methods such as "La Silla Vacia/The Empty Chair" in my role as vice president at a community college. In this regard, one of my responsibilities that gave me much satisfaction, was to interview all students who were at the point of being dismissed from the college for not maintaining either a minimum grade point average or because of lack of completion of a sufficient number of units with passing grades. (As you may recall, I was such a student because I failed at my first attempt to attend community college at Laney College in Oakland, California!).

Over and over, students communicated many personal doubts and emotional conflicts that placed psychological roadblocks in their ability to succeed in their studies at the college. Examples of this are that many students were fearful regarding whether or not they possessed the skills necessary to succeed in college, and, very often, many were overwhelmed by the emotional challenges of college as well as life in general with anxiety, depression, and feelings of shame in not having achieved success in school and life.

Students showed an interest in hearing about how I personally developed my ability to manage my emotions by doing Gestalt personal development work, and they often asked me to do "work" with them. I thought and thought about how I could do quick work with students to help them gain insights for how to effectively face the emotional and psychological challenges of college. I talked to Morgan Goodlander at the Gestalt Institute of San Francisco, and he supported me to develop a simplified counseling approach that would use the basic concepts and methods of Gestalt therapy, but from an educational perspective of "teaching" students how to better understand and face their emotional challenges through Gestalt principles and practice. Thus, "Gestalt Educational Counseling" (GEC) was born.

What was born was a Gestalt-oriented psychological intervention that I have used with a countless number of students and community groups in and around Oakland and across the nation for over twenty-five years. Also, what was born was a chapter in a book called "Crossing Cultures in Gestalt Therapy: Gestalt Educational Counseling," published by the Gestalt Institute Press of New Orleans. Along with this publication, what also was forming within me was an idea of recruiting others to use GEC with community college students and Latin@ community members. This work of mine reflects the strength of my *"Latinoness"* in the U.S.A., that is, a compassion for feeling the hurt of others and wanting to improve the sociopsychological experience of others.

My idea was to establish a Gestalt Institute of Oakland. The goal of wanting to start a Gestalt Institute in Oakland has proven very challenging for me, with some lows and highs related to success. One example of a low point in this endeavor is when I attempted to orient the counseling faculty at Vista College to the power of Gestalt work to support personal counseling work with students. I met resistance, which too often has been the case with many counseling professionals. "You can use this with students, but keep it away from us," was the response from the majority of counselors at my college.

I didn't give up. Instead, I have continued this effort over the years in my consulting and volunteer community work, and have had some success in training counselors to consider using GEC in their work with students. One such effort was with the counseling faculty at Del Mar College, a community college in Corpus Christi, Texas. Here is a quote from one of the counselors who attended a three-day training in the use of GEC: "The most important thing I learned today is the intense power of the process [GEC] for change. As the leader allowed participants to fully feel the moment and pushed them to go with the feeling even if it felt awkward or uncomfortable . . . what I would like to learn more about is really just watching and experiencing the process. I'm focusing my attention on the skills used by the leader in facilitating the process." Key in the latter phrase is "fully feel the moment." In many ways, Gestalt personal development involves the experience of being able to stay with one's difficult feelings until a balance in our experience of feelings is achieved. More about this soon.

Related to wanting to start a Gestalt Institute of Oakland, a goal of mine has been to mentor students of color who want to be psychologists by introducing them and training them in Gestalt practices. While I have yet to achieve the vision of starting a Gestalt Institute in Oakland, I definitely have introduced hundreds, if not thousands, of persons to Gestalt personal development methods and practices. One example of this is the work I have done with Ms. Yuselin Martinez, a young Latina Marriage Family Therapy (MFT) graduate student at San Francisco State University whom I began to mentor when she was a student in the Peralta Community College District.

Yuselin does community work in Catholic churches with Latin@ community members in and around Oakland. She has called on me many times to do Gestalt work with community groups wherein I teach and do group work in Spanish related to Gestalt personal development theory and methods related to personal growth, and use the method of *"La Silla Vacia"* to show individuals how they can infuse more strength and peace in living their lives. I have also repeated this in trainings for Bay Area Women Against Rape (BAWAR), also in Oakland (only six blocks from where my mama raised my brother and me), where I have taught Gestalt principles and practices to volunteer Latino@ peer counselors who work at BAWAR. Finally, I have done Gestalt personal development work with hundreds of students during my work as a psychology professor and administrator at Merritt College, Berkeley City College, and San Francisco State University.

Developing an Educationally-Focused Gestalt Counseling Approach

My goal consistently has been to develop a Gestalt

personal development approach that is more understandable and accessible to mama's "*nuestro proximo*," to individuals and groups that do not have ready access to psychological resources to support their personal and psychological growth. In this regard, I am reminded of the words of Amado Padilla, who asserted that Latinos need education first, then counseling, and finally, therapy, if they so desire to help themselves face challenges to psychological development in their lives. I think I have been very successful in developing an approach, Gestalt Educational Counseling, which I see as practical and accessible to persons who are beginning their journey to define and support their psychological uniqueness: first, education, then counseling, and finally, therapy, if necessary, or if a person so chooses.

What I call Gestalt Educational Counseling is based on an orientation of psychological education to which I was introduced while completing my doctoral studies at the University of Minnesota, Minneapolis (U of M). The orientation was that of psychoeducational studies, which was a movement that was led in great part by educational and counseling psychologists at the U of M who championed the importance of making psychoeducational studies an integral part of K-12 education. I am a product of this vision, and my work in bringing GEC to inner city communities reflects the vision of psychoeducational studies as well as my mother's vision of "helping our fellow human beings- *nuestro proximo*."

I initially developed the use of Gestalt methods of personal development to assist community college students, and especially, students of color, to gain knowledge about how they could learn to take more responsibility for their efforts to succeed in college: (1) by becoming aware of how their childhood psychological legacies may have affected their present-day efforts to take on the emotional and intellectual challenges of college and life; and (2) how they can assume greater control and responsibility of their achievement efforts in college by using the Gestalt methods of "self-support."

Importantly, in the latter part of this chapter, you will see a shift in my use of GEC from a more general to specific approach. I did this because I wanted to ensure that persons' initial exposure to Gestalt methods would result in a clear understanding of both the theory and methods of Gestalt personal growth work. My initial approach involved teaching about Gestalt concepts of personal development and doing what I would call "unstructured" Gestalt work and counseling with students and others. However, in time, I further developed the specificity of GEC so as to more directly teach persons how blocks in their psychological growth were primarily a result of their Childhood Legacy of negative learning.

Initially, I used GEC as a method of counseling that combined teaching the principles of Gestalt personal development along with directly experiencing Gestalt methods of personal growth. At the center, my approach assumed that learning the ideas and concepts of Gestalt along with actual experience doing Gestalt work was an important prerequisite for underrepresented, ethnically diverse community college students to be more effective and successful in college.

From a Latin@ perspective, an important aspect of GEC, directly in line with the idea of teaching students how to benefit from Gestalt counseling work, is the notion of the counselor modeling interpersonal openness about his or her personal growth challenges. This approach is in line with

Sidney Jourard's 1964 book, "Transparent Self," with the conception of counselors facilitating growth in clients by presenting "a transparent self," a person who is open about his or her own developmental challenges, and who supports others to open up and share themselves as part of the process of growing and becoming a more effective person. This interpersonal openness approach is also essential to supporting growth in ethnically diverse persons because it recognizes that students of color often enter community college having had many negative experiences in education that have resulted in a damaging lack of trust about how sincere and committed counselors, teachers, and administrators are regarding caring about and wanting to support their success. Also, interpersonal openness by the counselor is consistent with the Latin@ value of "*personalismo*," which means that Latin@s value being personable with others, that is, liking to have a warm interpersonal relationship.

A counselor who shares his/her "self" with students of color supports and encourages these students to trust the counselor, thereby increasing the students' willingness to open up and share their personal doubts and insecurities, which very often are based on hurtful childhood experiences where interpersonal mistrust became a way of facing the world. Achieving openness can then help students do the difficult personal development work needed to become self-aware for how they need to develop to be more effective in college and life in general.

Beyond emphasizing the importance of expressing interpersonal openness as a way of developing psychological strength, Gestalt methods focus on becoming aware of what I would call the "organismic process of personal growth." This means that biologically each of us is an organism that needs to function in a unified way, and that the best way to achieve this is to be united or integrated as a person in how we think, feel, and act. What I have taken from Gestalt therapy is how to develop a basic awareness for how as individuals we can be more unified in our approach to life and therefore take more charge of our psychological growth.

Referring back to Chapter 1, "Key Gestalt Principles Related to Personal Development and Professional Growth," the central approach of GEC is the teaching of the phases of the "Gestalt Cycle of Experience," as well as taking persons through the actual experience of Gestalt personal development through use of *"La Silla Vacia."* Conceptually, GEC emphasizes the importance of becoming aware and addressing the "internal split" that exists in many students of color between "I can," versus "I can't." The "I cans" are the "embodied" beliefs and feelings of hope and resilience of students of color that they can succeed in college, and the "I cant's" are the "embodied" beliefs that becoming a successful student is not achievable.

The "I can's" for me come from the support and love that family members and others give to the student, as well as from the natural, biological drive that we all have to complete ourselves in positive ways. The "I cant's" come from negative childhood emotional experiences, both in and outside of school, which too often leave debilitating psychological effects that produce shame and doubt about one's ability to achieve success in college and life.

Chapter 7

Case Scenarios –
Community College Students Learning Gestalt
(Adapted from Gestalt Educational Counseling
in "Crossing Cultures in Therapy," 2005)

Lack of Self-Support and Gestalt
Educational Counseling (GEC)

I now want to present examples of GEC interventions to show how this counseling approach can be used with students who come from backgrounds that subject them to more difficult challenges of adjustment in college in comparison to students who enter college with a greater amount of built-up psychological self-support, as well as knowledge and skills-readiness for college. In these counseling scenarios, there are two basic issues presented by students. One is their lack of "self-support" about belief in their ability to succeed in college. The other basic concern is that there is a split within the personality of many of the students between a "hopeful self" and a "doubtful or negating self."

Importantly, this split often results from actual negative experiences that students have had in their educational histories, many times centered in instances when teachers, counselors, and others in the school system were not sufficiently supportive of learning challenges experienced by students, or were negating or overly critical toward students. Non-supportive family-related experiences also negatively affect students' reservoir of strengths to handle the challenges of college. In summary, rather than a sense of hope and strength, students carried with them from their childhood feelings of shame and doubt regarding their ability to succeed in academic pursuits.

The Four Components of Gestalt
Educational Counseling (GEC)

Gestalt Educational Counseling has four component parts. These components address informational, relational, and personal development concerns that hamper learning that many students of color bring with them into their academic pursuits. First, to provide students with useful information about possible difficulties associated with attending college, the counselor introduces different examples of the intellectual, emotional, and behavioral challenges that students can face in college. This information is intended to clarify for students that the challenges they face as learners are not uniquely theirs, but common and normal to many students. One major example of a challenge that students face in beginning college is to objectively assess their skills readiness for doing college work, which means facing the challenging truth about the need to do difficult intellectual and emotional work to catch up to where one should be.

Along with information about typical personal and academic challenges faced by many students, the counselor addresses how counseling can help students face their difficulties. A key relational strategy is that the counselor shares personal challenges he or she experienced when attending college. A big challenge that I bring up is that throughout college, students may face self-doubt regarding the ability to master learning tasks that initially seem too difficult and even impossible to learn, e.g., understanding assigned readings, difficult math problems, organizing how to write a research paper, etc. Personally, I share instances when I had to get help from others and had to work very hard to overcome my personal doubts about my skills and ability to learn.

The second step of GEC involves the counselor sharing experienced emotional difficulties and how counseling has been beneficial for successfully handling academic and personal growth challenges. For example, I have shared with students that at one point in my doctoral study, I became very anxious, tense, and filled with fear of failure, so much so that I was unable to focus my mind and body on the task of writing my dissertation. I literally at one point couldn't move! I share that I was able to make it through this challenge with the loving help of others (remember Leroy Gardner at the University of Minnesota?), although not as effectively as I think I could have if I would have done Gestalt personal development work. I also share that through Gestalt counseling, I learned how to be more in charge of my personal growth. This second step is a combination of informational, relational, and conceptual aspects of GEC.

Third, the counselor introduces GEC and specific Gestalt concepts for how students can improve their psychological strengths related to difficult emotions faced in college. In Chapter 2 of this book, I have described these concepts. By way of example, students are told that Gestalt counseling is a way of learning to understand and manage emotions, to become more aware of one's emotional life and its relationship to negative and non-supportive childhood experiences, and to become a person who "can identify what he or she wants and how to go about getting it" (Nevis, 1987). This step is primarily conceptual in that I am teaching about the meaning behind Gestalt personal development counseling.

The fourth step in GEC is when the counselor conducts individual or group Gestalt Educational Counseling, again, a combination of counseling and teaching, so that students experience the power of Gestalt counseling methods, and at the same time learn through instruction from the counselor how Gestalt counseling methods relate to personal growth, and that the methods can be used on an ongoing basis to increase effective participation in college and life.

The instruction part of GEC involves the counselor using "teaching moments" while doing work with students to clarify the process of psychological challenge and growth from a Gestalt perspective. In my initial use and development of GEC, I would do what I would call spontaneous and unstructured Gestalt counseling work, much like the psychological group work I had experienced at the Gestalt Institute of San Francisco. This work focuses on a person's immediate felt experience to arrive at "growth points" where the person is tested by having to "stay with" and learn self-support in facing challenging emotions.

Gestalt Counseling Group Workshops with Ethnically Diverse College Students

From 1988 to 2019, I provided counseling to many students who were subject to dismissal from college. I did this as part of my duties as Associate Dean of Undergraduate Studies at San Francisco State University and as Vice President of Student Services at Vista College/Berkeley City College, and as a psychology teacher and mentor to community college students at Merritt College in Oakland. I also used GEC methods as part of my consulting and counseling work with well-established academic support programs in higher education, such as the Educational and Opportunity Programs and Services (EOPS), Puente, Math, Engineering and Science Achievement (MESA) Summer Leadership Program, and San Francisco State University's National Institute of Health, Bridges to Health Sciences Baccalaureate Program.

The settings of the GEC program interventions were varied, but generally consisted of either individual counseling sessions or daylong group meetings for first-generation, low-income underrepresented students enrolled in academic success and leadership programs. The primary goal of the GEC workshops was to support students to be better prepared intellectually, emotionally, and behaviorally to handle challenging academic majors, including engineering, chemistry, physics, and pre-health preparation (medicine, pharmacy, dentistry, etc.). As a general overview of GEC, the format followed in workshops, though abbreviated here, will be used as a means of describing how I conducted GEC in a group setting.

Understanding and Supporting Self When Doubt, Shame, and Fear Hamper Academic Success

In the initial part of the workshops, students are introduced to the notion that every individual has the potential to meet the diverse challenges of college. As a way of inspiring students to believe in their inborn ability to learn, I act out the experience of an infant learning to walk. I get down on all fours on the floor mimicking a child who is learning to walk. I try to communicate how learning to walk for an infant is a totally novel experience, and that each movement, from steadying self by grabbing hold of an available surface to letting go of that surface and having to steady the self on shaky legs, is a potentially threatening experience fraught with a mixture of doubt and apprehension, as well as hope and excitement.

I ask students the following question: "How many times does a thirteen-month-old child fall down when learning to walk before he or she gives up learning how to walk?" The answer, of course, is that the child falls down countless times, and, in a very natural way, never gives up. The students understand this instantly, because they observe without being prompted that, "it's part of our nature to walk," and that, "children have something inside which makes them keep trying," and that, "it's exciting to keep trying to walk until you achieve your goal!" Here I introduce the word intrinsic to emphasize that we all have within us an inborn (*intrinsic*) and natural strength to learn. Also, I connect this example of learning to walk and not giving up, as analogous/similar to taking tests in college and failing (falling down), and how we all have in us the inborn, intrinsic ability to stand up and keep trying! Nevertheless, I always add, "Too often very many of us have learned to give up rather than continually trying to pick ourselves up and learn how to re-do our "mis-takes" and become effective.

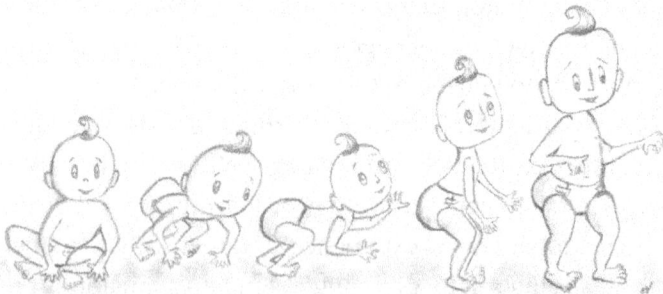

In learning to walk, a child constantly works on the "mistakes" that are natural to learning

The following is another anecdote that I use to inspire students to be aware of how negative early learning experiences can get in the way of their belief in their ability to face the challenges of difficult learning situations: "If you went into a kindergarten classroom and asked for all those students who could sing to raise their hands, how many hands would go up?" The answer given by students, generally, is that almost all the hands in the class would be raised. I then follow this with a similar question about how many high school seniors would raise their hands to the same question. Students answer that only a few high school seniors, if any, would raise their hands to such a question.

A discussion then follows that there are many people in our society who experience our schools as "fear factories," where students learn to "compare and despair" about their ability to be skillful in comparison to others. Specific to ethnic minority students, Claude Steele, in his book "Whistling Vivaldi," has named this phenomenon "stereotype threat," wherein many students of color spend more time worrying about how they compare to other students in their abilities, rather than focusing on paying attention to and completing the learning task at hand.

A question I ask related to the experience of "compare and despair" is the following: "In elementary school, what do other children often do in a classroom when a child makes a mistake?" The answer is that other students often laugh and snicker, which embarrasses and shames a child, and too often leads to fear of learning and to comparing oneself as not being as smart as the other children. Sadly, this too often occurs with second-language learners.

Going back to the infant learning to walk, I make the point that a child learning to walk does not stop from continuing to try by saying negative statements to self when making missteps. For example, the infant does not think, "I sure look stupid falling down!" or "I must really be dumb falling down!" or "I'll never be able to learn how to walk!" "No," I insist. "Negative self-statements such as the latter sadly are learned in the process of growing up, too often from feedback that is given to individuals by misguided family members, peers, counselors, or teachers who incorrectly criticize a child's mistakes, too often resulting in persons internalizing a negative, criticizing self whenever mistakes are made."

Emphasizing that We All Can Right Ourselves in Difficult Situations and Achieve Success

At this point in the workshop a discussion ensues with students emphasizing that each of them has within the drive to move forward in powerful ways toward cherished goals, much like the child learning to stand and walk. Here I discuss the following quotes: "Everybody is born unique, but most of us die copies," and "Get better not bitter," and "It is our birthright to achieve completeness." The discussion then centers on how to recapture the strength and drive to learn to be as effective as possible in our lives, a strength naturally possessed by the developing child in so many of his/her efforts, or "how to support self to keep going when things get tough."

I then move to modeling interpersonal openness where my goal is to emphasize that it is human to err, and that we must learn to support and not reject ourselves when we do not measure up to our or other's expectations. Here, I emphasize the importance of "*personalismo*" or "interpersonal openness," and being part of a community (*comunidad*) as factors that support our psychological growth. I share personal experiences from my own life regarding challenges to my growth. In this instance, I share having come from a broken home with a very abusive, negative, and frightening father, and having been separated from my mother for two years at the age of seven after my mother had divorced my father and could not keep her children with her because she was too poor.

Along with this, I share my fearful learning history stemming from coming from a welfare family, and where my mother only had a sixth-grade education and only spoke Spanish so could not guide my development of English skills. I share that my early life experiences translated into me becoming diffident (modest or shy because of a lack of self-confidence) about myself as a potential learner, because I compared myself to others in society whom I felt came from better families or who were more skillful or smarter, especially non-Latin@ whites.

As a final part of this time of personal sharing, I also share some of my more significant later challenges in college wherein I often felt very fearful, as when I flunked out of Laney Community College or when I became really scared and felt that I could not continue toward finishing my doctorate. I conclude this portion of my communication to students by sharing with them how Gestalt counseling methods helped me to be more psychologically effective in facing the learning and emotional challenges of life, and then how Gestalt personal development counseling helped me to learn to breathe and not tense up and trust myself in difficult learning situations.

Gestalt Group Work with Students to Help
Them Develop Greater Emotional Strength

In the next part of doing GEC in a group workshop, students are introduced to key Gestalt concepts that define how to strengthen our psychological selves, ideas that will benefit them as they experience Gestalt counseling. Specifically, I teach them about Joseph Zinker's 1977 book, "The Creative Process in Gestalt Therapy," which outlines a process -the Gestalt Cycle of Experience- for how individuals can learn to successfully experience or face emotionally challenging life events.

The Cycle proceeds from (1) SENSATION — the experience of body sensations to (2) AWARENESS — being aware that with our sensations we are having a "felt reaction" to our life experience — a sensory response that signals that there is something we want or need from life, to (3) MOBILIZATION OF ENERGY — when we naturally respond to our sensations by beginning to mobilize our energy to do something about the dissatisfaction we are experiencing to (4) ACTION — taking action or experimenting with different ways of responding to a situation that causes dissatisfaction to (5) CONTACT — or having an experience where one comes in contact with oneself having the experience of meeting one's needs to (6) ASSIMILATION — integrating or assimilating the learning experience itself into one's overall sense of being a unique human being, and finally, to (7) WITHDRAWAL — withdrawal from the experience of a challenging life event because it is completed. Following withdrawal from challenging events, we move on to other cycles of experience associated with whatever life circumstance emerges (emergencies) as most important to us.

In the GEC workshops, students are further introduced to the notion that individuals can stop themselves from going through the "Gestalt Cycle of Experience" because they do not have enough "self-support" to work through difficult emotions experienced in each phase of the cycle. I repeatedly emphasize that this lack of self-support is learned as a result of negative past life experiences, especially in childhood, wherein students were not sufficiently supported by family, relatives, teachers, etc. or were de-stabilized and learned "non-self-support" because of sexual, physical, or psychological trauma.

Students learn about specific Gestalt "self-support" concepts and methods to be able to understand and do their own personal development work. One concept is that of "Organismic Self-regulation," which is a concept initially developed by Kurt Goldstein in his book "The Organism" that gave evidence that each person has the inborn (intrinsic) ability to support self during difficult life circumstances. This concept emphasizes that an effective person is one who can continually move forward and learn more ways of supporting self to face and work through difficult emotional trials. Similarly, the importance of accepting, staying with, and focusing on developing greater awareness of one's physical reactions to situations is reinforced to support the person to be more in touch with their unique visceral (felt body experience) emotional reactions to life events.

Finally, a very helpful Gestalt concept is the principle of polarity, which introduces the notion that individuals split themselves into a warring splits in personality- Perls' "Top Dog versus Underdog self" - that leads to becoming *stuck* in difficult life situations, because the individual cannot resolve the inner war between a supporting self (usually the

"Underdog") and a doubting or negating self (the "Top Dog), and, therefore, finds it difficult to move in a unified and energized way toward a desired goal.

Introduction to "*La Silia Vacia*" - Unifying the Personality

At this point in the workshop, I introduce students to The Gestalt Empty Chair Technique or "*La Silla Vacia*," which uses two chairs to pit warring aspects of self that require resolution and integration. Resolution involves helping the individual become aware of the two aspects of self, and how these polar opposites cause indecision, confusion, and doubt, and require uniting or integrating so as to make a person a more functional whole. Here, students put one of the warring parts of self in one chair and the contradicting aspect of self in the other chair. I then assist them to act out a dialogue between the conflicting parts within themselves while shuttling back and forth between the two chairs. This counseling method helps clarify at what point within that dialogue or conflict the person is stuck or is having an "impasse" related to their psychological growth.

Students soon learn that this method uncovers long-held "unfinished business," very often related to negative experiences with significant people in their development (recall me with the VP at SFSU), which has become part of the personality (has been introjected) as non-supportive emotions and beliefs toward the self. Students consequently learn that becoming more aware of these internal conflicts will allow them to (1) let go of these conflicts by becoming aware of how the conflicts are internalized and expressed in their physical selves (we are some<u>body</u>), and (2) learn to take responsibility and experiment with making more effective thinking, feeling, and behavior choices (experiments) when trying to resolve present-day psychological challenges.

When introducing students to the benefits of Gestalt work, the key for me is to discuss how I learned to work through difficult challenges by using Gestalt methods to free myself from behavioral, cognitive, and emotional habits related to fear, shame, and doubt that I had developed in myself as a child. As I have said, I share concrete examples of how my past negative learning within my family and from some of my childhood school experiences resulted in my initial inability to support myself through difficult challenges in college. After the short discussion of the Gestalt Cycle of Experience and related concepts, I ask for volunteers to do Gestalt work on issues related to their inability to face academic challenges. In this regard, I have always been amazed as to how eager students are to do this work. I always see in them a courageous energy to learn how to improve their psychological self.

What now follows are some anecdotes of the work I have done with students. These sessions involved students who were asked to share challenges that they were experiencing in college as well as ways that they wanted to learn to improve success in their studies. As the students took turns speaking about difficulties with their studies, I would invite some of them to do individual Gestalt chair work in front of the group. Of course, two important norms of these groups were that the sharing of students was voluntary and confidential.

Students Learning Gestalt in
Academic Achievement Workshops

In this section I share the beginnings of what I call Gestalt Educational Counseling (GEC), including group and individual work, again, a combination of teaching about Gestalt and doing general Gestalt work. When I say general work, I mean that beyond teaching a little about Gestalt personal development concepts, I mainly used the counseling approach I learned at the Gestalt Institute. This approach involved doing empty chair work to help the students develop an awareness of the connection between their emotional selves, the physical manifestation of their emotions, and how their emotions can block their growth.

I also aimed at teaching students how to learn to calm their anxieties by staying with their emotions to the point of being able to support themselves (learn self-support) to think and act more effectively regarding their psychological challenges. What follows are examples of work with students. The student names are fictitious and not connected to the actual name of participants. Following this section, I will introduce how I further developed my use of Gestalt counseling with students and community groups.

SERETA: Learning "Self-Support" to
Better Handle the Study of Chemistry

The first student to speak up was Sereta, a twenty-year-old African American female. She complained of not doing as well in her science coursework as she would like. After some questioning, I determined that Sereta had gotten a D grade in an introduction to chemistry course, and consequently that she was feeling insecure toward pursuing her science-related major. Also, Sereta complained of "not being able to support" herself enough to stick with very challenging science coursework. I noted that Sereta was not breathing very deeply, she was holding herself in a very tense and tight manner, and her eyes were downcast.

I decided to work through what I saw in Sereta as a split or polarity in her approach to handling her problem between wanting to go forward, yet feeling a lack of confidence and positive energy to move forward. I asked Sereta if she would be willing to try empty chair work. Recall that a polarity or split in one's personality happens when a person is at odds within themself as to how to respond to a personal challenge, with one end of the polarity often being disparaging, and the other end of the polarity usually being more constructive, yet reflecting, as in this case, Sereta's doubting self. The end result is usually a split in the personality where the individual cannot think, feel, and act in an integrated or unified manner to handle psychological challenges. My hope for Sereta was that the empty chair experience would allow her to become more aware of the conflict between self-support and non-support by shuttling back and forth between the two chairs, while acting out and experiencing the associated feelings of the two sides of her psychological split.

After Sereta agreed to participate in this Gestalt counseling strategy, I asked her to sit in one of the two chairs where she would act out that part of herself that needed support (Need Support) to manage the challenging task of studying chemistry. In the other chair, Sereta would act out that part of herself that was unable to support (Unable to Support) herself. The following is part of the dialogue that took place during this Gestalt counseling session:

Need support: (Spoken to the chair with not enough strength to offer support to the weak self) "I can't do this without your support; it's too scary. I need your help."

Dr. Rivas: At this point, I asked Sereta to change the word "it's" to "I" in order to more directly experience the feeling (scary) to which Sereta was alluding, e.g., "I am too scary." Owning an experience as "I" versus "it" is important because from a Gestalt perspective each person is the creator of his or her experience. When Sereta says "I am scary," she is acknowledging that in great part she is creating her scariness. Yes, the study of chemistry is difficult for her, but the "scariness" comes from her unique reaction to the study of chemistry. At this point, I asked Sereta to switch from the "need for support chair" to the "unable to support chair." In this new position, she was to respond to the request for help.

Unable to Support: In this chair, Sereta looked down and seemed not to want to respond to the request for support that she had just made from the other chair. I could see that Sereta's body in the non-support chair was tense and tight with frustration. I waited quietly for Sereta to say or do something, noticing that she seemed unable to look up or to take any action. This patient waiting is necessary and useful for two reasons: (1) the waiting gives Sereta an opportunity to gather her strength to respond to the request, and (2) waiting also allows Sereta to stay with her reaction to a request for support from the "unable to support self" position.

This waiting can be very stressful, and so the waiting allows Sereta to learn in her body that she doesn't necessarily need to turn away from the feeling of self-doubt or fear, and that she can "hold herself in the experience of difficult emotions." Also, waiting for a response also acknowledges that each person has the inner strength (Organismic Self-regulation) to handle their emergencies. If the counselor sees that the person is not holding their strength well, an experiment can be initiated, which is the "action" part of the "Gestalt Cycle of Experience" to help the student better handle the difficult psychological moment. In my interaction with Sereta, I then asked her whether she had heard the request for support.

Unable to Support: Sereta answered "Yes."

Dr. Rivas: I asked Sereta in the Unable to Support Chair, "Do you think you can try to respond to the request for support?" At this point, Sereta looked up, and in a tired and tense manner said the following:

Unable to Support: "No, I can't support you."

Dr. Rivas: I suggested that Sereta switch back to the chair identified as "Need for Support."

I then asked: "How did you feel when you heard the rejection to your request for support? What was your feeling then?"

Sereta said she felt confused and hurt, and then she began to tear up and then to cry. I moved closer to her and placed my hand on her shoulder while she cried. This simple action on my part is an example of "Other Support," and, indeed, is experienced as a strengthening physical support from the counselor, especially if the counselor has established a trusting, open, and supportive rapport with the person seeking help. I then asked Sereta to switch to the "Unable to Support" chair.

After Sereta switched chairs, I inquired about what she felt watching Sereta cry in the "Need for Support" chair.

Unable to Support: "I feel tense. I don't know. I guess I feel some tension in my shoulders and in my arms and I hesitate but want to reach out to her."

Dr. Rivas: I asked Sereta, "Can you share with Sereta who needs support that you find it difficult to reach out to her in support, and that you feel that hesitancy in your arms and legs?"

Unable to support: "I find it hard to want to reach out to help you, and I feel that in my arms and legs."

Dr. Rivas: I find that this is an important part of Gestalt empty chair work, that is, for the person to own and express their true and honest experience of their feelings. I think this helps build true awareness of the physical and psychological experience of the self.

Asking Sereta to now move back to the "Need for Support" chair, I then wondered aloud to her what she felt while listening to the Sereta in the "Unable to Support" chair. Sereta answered that she felt frustrated, but she felt a little okay because the "Unable to Support Sereta" was being a little honest about her lack of willingness to reach out to the "Need for Support Sereta." At this point, I noted that "The Need for Support Sereta" was holding her breath and not breathing very deeply. I also noted a look of intense emotion in her face. I wondered aloud whether this feeling of frustration and form of communication reminded her of any similar interactions that she had experienced with significant people in her life.

At this point, Sereta began to cry in a very intense way. This is an act that I have witnessed over and over with students (as well as myself in my own Gestalt personal development work), and to me it signals the experience and release of a long-held hurt and dissatisfaction within the person. I have learned to think of this experience as a "crisis of awareness." This crisis involves beginning to become aware of a past hurt or trauma that seemed overwhelming to the person when initially experienced. After allowing Sereta to cry for a number of minutes, I asked her if she could share what the present situation reminded her of from her past life. Sereta answered that she could. She then recounted a story of a time in her life when she was eleven. A very sad event occurred in her family, and Sereta was not adequately supported to understand what had occurred nor to understand the sadness, hurt, and loneliness associated with the experience. Sereta also shared how a key family member had been unable to offer care and support to her at that time, and, in fact, had talked very little to Sereta about the event.

Dr. Rivas speaking to Sereta in the "Need for Support" chair: I now asked Sereta if she had wanted support from her family member at that time; also, what she had felt during that experience. Sereta answered that she very much wanted to talk to her family about how she was confused and sad related to what had occurred in her life and how much she needed care and support from her family. I then went on to ask Sereta if her relationship with her family had improved since this sad childhood event. Sereta answered that her relationship with her family around the event had remained pretty much the same.

Dr. Rivas: At this point, I inquired of the group members whether someone from the group would come up and sit in the "Unable to Support" chair and offer Sereta the support she needed. A Caucasian woman was the first to volunteer, although an older African American man and a Latina young woman soon after also volunteered. Though strongly inclined to choose the African American male, I chose the

Caucasian woman because she had jumped out of her chair and had expressed a strong willingness to offer support to Sereta.

My choice was based on me surveying the environment which was multicultural, and deciding to support the "environment of the moment" that seemed to call for accepting what I perceived as a genuine request from the Caucasian woman to offer support to Sereta. I imagined similar perceptions on the part of the diverse members of the group, so I asked the volunteer student to offer her support to Sereta, almost as if she was Sereta's family member. The following is the dialogue that ensued.

Volunteer in the Unable to Support Chair: "I know that I have not given you the support that you need, but I want you to know that I love you very much and that I very much want to support your hurt and confusion."

The volunteer then embraced Sereta, and both of the students cried. I allowed this encounter to continue for a few minutes, again, being patient and allowing the situation to be felt and experienced as completely as possible. This waiting is important because the person or persons (in this case two persons, but really the entire group of persons, because they are also experiencing the interaction in a vicarious way) are allowed enough time to feel and integrate the interaction (make part of their body and mind).

After a moment or two, I asked, "Sereta, what are you now feeling?" Sereta, in the Need for Support Chair, responded by saying that she felt calm and peaceful. I asked Sereta where in her body she was feeling calm and peaceful, and Sereta said in her heart. I also noted out loud that Sereta was breathing in a more relaxed and deep manner.

Dr. Rivas: At this point I ended the chair work, and

asked Sereta to take a seat next to me and to face the group. Next, I began soliciting from Sereta what insights she had gained from this Gestalt counseling session. Sereta said that she had not known how much the lack of support at a key time in her childhood had affected her. Also, she said that she needed to learn how to better support herself when she became confused or hurt during her studies. I then invited Sereta to walk around the group and choose students to look in the eye and say, "I need to learn to support myself better when I get confused or hurt regarding my studies." Sereta did this, and two of the students she chose were the African American man and the Latina who had initially volunteered to play the role of the caring family member.

As for the African American man, he told Sereta that she could always count on him to support her whenever she doubted herself. He also told Sereta that he thought she was a strong woman who would succeed in achieving her goals in college. He also thanked her for having the strength to share this difficult experience with the group.

An interesting side point here is that research at the University of California, Berkeley, found that African American students (in the study it was African American males), to their detriment, often isolate themselves and study alone more than other groups of students. Back to the group.

The Latina stood and asked Sereta if she could hug her, to which Serena said yes. At the same time, the Latina group member said that she experienced Sereta's challenges similar to her challenges and that she had learned that she, like Sereta, needed to practice loving and supporting herself during challenging and stressful times.

As part of the teaching part of GEC, while working with Sereta, I, at different points in the session, introduced important Gestalt concepts, such as the observation that barely breathing can indicate not supporting self or that splits in one's personality may lead to moments of impasse, to being stuck in a position of inaction or inability to act in an effective manner, that is, to move along the cycle from sensation, to awareness, to mobilization of energy, etc. Also, I shared with students that often the inability to resolve our present-day challenges are connected to past life traumas, many from childhood, wherein we learned non-supportive ways of facing difficult feelings, thoughts, and behaviors. In this case, Sereta had long ago learned to shut down her need for "self-support" as well as "other support."

This example of Gestalt counseling with a group of multicultural community college students exemplifies how Gestalt methods can be used in a practical way to help students understand the "psychology of attending college." Specifically, in the case of Sereta, we find a student who because of a significant past experience with a significant family member, did not learn sufficiently how to support herself in a situation where confusion, doubt, and fear combined to lessen her ability to support herself in the face of a difficult challenge. Importantly, this lessening of psychological strength was fixed in bodily reactions to stress that prevented positive action toward resolving challenges.

Sereta and her groupmates saw the counselor use a Gestalt strategy of allowing Sereta to dialogue with different parts of herself that were in conflict regarding whether or not she could support herself to face a confusing and fearful situation in her college experience. Sereta learned that this was an internal dialogue that she had not sufficiently been addressing in her life. Through the "La *Silla Vacia*" experience, Sereta learned to respond to life challenges in a more

unified, integrated way, a way that was more complete
wherein she did not hide from difficult emotions, where she
could feel her fears and doubts and not move away from
them, and, at the same time to understand her emotional
self in a way that allowed for improving her way of thinking, feeling, and acting.

Sereta learned about the importance of holding and supporting herself when experiencing difficult emotions. On
practical level, Sereta said that she was going to practice
"self-support" by seeking help from teachers, tutors, etc.,
when needed, rather than distancing herself from the negative feelings of doubt and shame that she often felt during
such times. I knew that this would translate to more positive
energy in Sereta's body to "lean forward" into difficult experiences.

CARMEN: Learning "Self-Support" to Continue Engineering, though Initially Receiving an F Grade in Physics

The second example of Gestalt Educational Counseling
applied to community college students from diverse backgrounds is with a student named Carmen. Participating in a
different group from Sereta, Carmen, a twenty-one-year-old
Latina, complained of feeling discouraged in college because
of her poor grades. I inquired about Carmen's performance,
and she informed me that she had earned a B in chemistry,
but had failed her first physics course. This grade of F
weighed heavily on Carmen. Her shoulders felt heavy, her
arms felt tense, and her stomach was painful. She very discouraged about continuing her studies in engineering.

I asked Carmen if she would be willing to do some
Gestalt work regarding her poor physics grade. Carmen

accepted, and I set up two chairs, one for Carmen to act out her discouraging thoughts, feelings, and behaviors related to earning an F in physics, and the other for Carmen to speak to her discouraged self as if she were the physics course.

I want to discuss how I, as a Gestalt-trained counselor, went about choosing what aspects of Carmen's problem to put in each of the chairs. With Sereta, the choice was straightforward. In one chair was Sereta's "Need for Support," and the other was her being "Unable to Support" herself. With Carmen, the conceptual orientation was the same, self-support versus lack of self-support, so I put in one chair, "Unable to Support Self," Carmen's "feeling discouraged or unable to support self because of the failing grade." In the "Lack of Support" chair, I asked Carmen to act out the "physics course with the grade of F." In short, Carmen's "acting out" the failed physics course would allow her to become keenly aware about what thoughts and feelings she was experiencing with regard to having taken and failed physics.

Carmen's response to the F grade in the physics course, the lack of self-support chair, I hypothesized, was in great part an internalized (the term in Gestalt is *introjected*) way of approaching a difficult psychological "emergency" that was possibly learned in childhood when Carmen was faced with a challenging psychological experience for which she was not developmentally prepared and did not receive sufficient other-support, an emergency wherein she learned "lack of self-support" rather than "self-support." Carmen's possible learned childhood response of non-support, I have learned from repeated work with students from similar backgrounds, was internalized as the inability to support self in similar endeavors in the future.

Dr. Rivas: I first asked Carmen to sit in the Poor Physics Grade Chair and to share with me what she felt in that chair. Carmen said that she felt hopeless and discouraged. I then asked Carmen if she could request support from the "Tough Physics Course" chair. Here, you can see the beginnings of me formalizing a more teaching and structured Gestalt Educational Counseling approach. In this approach, I guide or take a more directive approach in offering help than what I had learned at the Gestalt Institute. I "experiment" or "try out" different statements with the person in each of the chair positions to essentially move the person to experience "self-support" and "non-self-support" positions.

"Unable to Support" discouraged self in response to physics course F grade: "I feel hopeless and discouraged," Carmen added. "And, I can't understand you." (Carmen's added statement is significant because the words were hers not mine, which means that they are figural (recall Figure/Ground) or very significant for her in facing the challenge of the F grade in physics).

Dr. Rivas: I then encouraged Carmen to switch chairs and to speak to the "Discouraged Carmen" from the "Tough Physics Course" chair.

Physics Course Chair (to discouraged Carmen): "I am too complex, and you'll never understand me, especially because you're too stubborn." (Carmen volunteered this entire statement).

Dr. Rivas: At this point, Carmen began to tear up. I then suggested she move from the "Poor Physics Grade" chair to the "Discouraged Carmen" chair. After doing this, Carmen became very emotional, so much so that she could not look up as she heaved and cried very strongly. I quietly watched her, allowing Carmen to thoroughly experience her emotions. After a couple of minutes, I asked Carmen if her interaction with the "Tough Physics Course" chair reminded her of any interactions with key people in her life. To this question, Carmen's crying became more intense.

I waited patiently for Carmen to feel her way into and through the painful emotions that she was remembering from the past and reliving in the present moment. After a short time, I wondered aloud whether Carmen would be willing to share who from a past encounter was coming to her mind in this present situation. Carmen softly revealed, "My aunt, who raised me, was always tough on me, and compared me negatively to my other younger cousins."

Dr. Rivas: I followed Carmen's disclosure by asking her if she was willing to put her aunt in the "Tough Physics Course" chair. She agreed. I then asked her to speak to the chair designated as her aunt.

Carmen: "You never support me; you always treat me like I am not important. All I ever want is your help, but you always turn your back on me."

Dr. Rivas: I then encouraged Carmen to switch to the aunt chair and to then respond to Carmen as if she were the substitute parent aunt.

Aunt: "I know that you don't like me because I compared you unfavorably to your cousins. You're always so stubborn and you never listen to me. You'll never be successful because you always want to do everything your way."

Dr. Rivas: At this point, I spoke to the group about what I thought might be happening in Carmen's present life. Specifically, I hypothesized, and admitted that this was only a hypothesis, that Carmen had possibly learned from her experience with her parent-aunt that some situations could not be figured out because the situation came down to Carmen holding her position of being stubborn versus giving in to another aspect of the situation that was not supportive. (Here you can see that I am attempting to teach at the same time that I am working with Carmen to become aware of how she may not sufficiently be supporting herself psychologically, as well as how she may approach changing her ways to handle this situation to add more "self-support.")

I then asked the group members if anyone saw the connection between Carmen's past experience and her present experience with physics. One member suggested that perhaps Carmen was being too stubborn in her approach to physics and that maybe she needed to be more flexible. I then asked Carmen if this feedback made sense to her. Carmen answered, "Yes." I, in turn, asked Carmen to elaborate. Carmen answered that she really tried hard to do well in physics, but that she had used the approach that had been effective for her in chemistry — intensive memorization. At this point, another group member asked Carmen if she had tried reading more basic physics books or using tutors to help her understand physics. Carmen said that she had not tried either of these alternatives.

At the end of this session, I asked Carmen what insights she had gleaned from the experience. Carmen acknowledged that she was possibly being inflexible in her way of approaching what she perceived as a very tough subject (similar to her tough parent-aunt) that was difficult to understand. This signaled to me that Carmen may have learned this approach in her childhood interactions with her unsupportive parent-aunt. She vowed to try the course again, but this time to reach out for help from those around her, including her professor, other students, and tutors, and that she would try the suggestion of reading basic physics textbooks. Carmen also volunteered that she clearly saw that she carried with her some intense unfinished (Gestalt "unfinished business") feelings from her interaction with her parent-aunt, whom Carmen felt had been hurtful and non-supportive toward her during a very difficult time in her life.

In this anecdote, you can see how the empty chair technique helps persons to clarify the possible origin of their present psychological challenge. Carmen's learning and internalizing of "non-support" in her interactions with her substitute parent had developed a way of responding to a difficult life situation with an inflexible attitude. As I review this anecdote from a previously published chapter, I can see that at that time in my work with students, I was using a more general Gestalt counseling model and not what I eventually developed as an updated Gestalt Educational Counseling method.

The major difference is that with the updated GEC, I use a more focused approach to support persons to move directly to childhood experiences that relate to current psychological challenges. Also, I have definitely become more directive in my work with persons so as to speed up the process of developing greater psychological awareness regarding possible childhood origins of current life's psychological challenges.

CARLOS: Learning "Self-support" to Overcome Feelings of Worthlessness

The third example of Gestalt counseling involves a counseling session with a twenty-three-year-old Chicano student who was completing his second year of community college. The difficulty that this student was facing was a deep hurt and shame regarding his current efforts in college. Specifically, Carlos was considering pursuing a different major than he had been studying in his first years of college. The problem was that this indecision about his major came on the heels of four to five years of abusing drugs as well as not advancing in college or a job. After two years of college, Carlos felt shame that he possibly was not going to follow through on a promise that he had made to his single-parent father who was funding Carlos' education.

After sharing my experience with Gestalt personal development work and reviewing some key concepts of Gestalt counseling, especially Self-support, the Gestalt Cycle of Experience, and use of The Empty Chair Technique to help persons clarify the dynamics of their psychological challenges, I began by asking Carlos to describe the feelings that he was experiencing. Carlos said that on top of shame, he was also experiencing a lot of anxiety regarding his present circumstances and toward his future. I asked him if he would like to try Gestalt counseling work to clarify his situation. He accepted. As noted, I previously shared with Carlos some background information on Gestalt counseling, including the end goal of Gestalt work, which was to help persons to be more aware of how their habitual negative thinking, feeling, and behaving was possibly an approach learned in childhood as a response to a difficult psychological challenge when he may have learned to not support himself effectively.

I next asked Carlos to play two roles, one being the anxious and ashamed part of himself, and, the other, that part of Carlos that was contemplating changing majors. I told

Carlos that the way he would play the two parts of himself was to alternate between two chairs, one which would be the anxious-ashamed part of Carlos and the other the part of Carlos that wanted to change majors. I asked Carlos to sit in one chair and first speak from the position of being anxious and ashamed and to share what he felt in that position.

Anxious-Ashamed Carlos: "Here I go again, messing up my life by not doing what I need to be doing!"

Dr. Rivas: "What are you feeling at this very moment?" I asked.

Anxious-Ashamed Carlos: Carlos answered, "It's the same old thing; I'm no good and am just proving that I'm worthless."

Dr. Rivas: "I want you to teach you to distinguish between the difference between thinking versus feeling, because this is an important part of what I want you to learn in your work with me. When I ask you to share what you're feeling, you respond with how you are thinking, "I'm worthless." This is a thought, but there is a feeling that accompanies this thought. What I would like you to do is to get in touch with how you are responding in your body, your feeling/emotional self, to this present psychological challenge. For example, you may feel pain in your head, neck, back, tightness in your legs, etc."

Anxious-Ashamed Carlos: "Thinking I'm worthless makes me feel like not breathing; makes me feel like closing my eyes to the world; makes me feel a shaky energy in my shoulders."

As I have become more skillful in the use of Gestalt counseling methods, I have learned to follow up on the energy that individuals report experiencing in their bodies. For example, I am struck in retrospect to how Carlos' shaky shoulders may possibly signal the beginnings of "Mobilization of Energy" from the Gestalt Cycle of Experience. The shaky shoulders, as I stay with this idea, might have signaled for Carlos a need to move to another way of holding and moving his body in response to the challenge of feeling worthless. Since the late nineties, I have learned to follow these "emerging figures" because they do indeed often signal an alternative way of acting on the part of the person doing Gestalt work, a way of acting that reflects "Organismic Self-Regulation," where the person's whole being is beginning to adapt and solve their psychological challenges. Back to Carlos.

Dr. Rivas: I then asked Carlos to switch chairs and be or act that part of self that was considering changing majors. Once Carlos switched chairs, I asked how he felt in the "Changing Major" chair. Carlos answered that he felt frustrated and scared. I then asked Carlos to speak to the "Anxious-Ashamed" chair from the Changing Major chair.

Changing Major: "I'm scared about you messing up my life again; scared about you taking me under again."

Dr. Rivas: I had Carlos switch to the "Anxious-Ashamed" chair, and to share what he was experiencing listening to the "Changing Major" chair. Carlos said that he felt lost and confused. I then asked him to speak from this feeling, which he seemed to be experiencing throughout his whole body.

Anxious-Ashamed: "I need your support; I'm scared and anxious and I don't know what to do."

Dr. Rivas: I asked Carlos to switch back to the "Changing Major" chair, and to share what he was thinking, feeling. Carlos in the "Changing Major" spoke to the "Anxious-Ashamed" chair.

Changing Major: "I don't want you in my life. I don't like you. I don't want to feel like you."

Dr. Rivas: This interaction clearly shows that Carlos was experiencing in himself "Lack of Self-support," even rejection of himself. Sensing that we might be nearing some sort of closure, I had Carlos review the dialogue that he had just carried out between two aspects of himself. I also prompted him to try changing the "you" statements in his dialogue to "I" or "me" statements. The following is an example.

Changing Major to Anxious-Ahamed: "I don't want you (me) in my life. I don't like you (me). I don't want to feel like you (me)."

When Carlos did this, he began to tear and cry. I then put my hand on Carlos' shoulder and asked him what he was thinking and feeling. Carlos told me that he could clearly see how bad he was treating himself and how much he was turning his back on that part of himself that really needed his support. Carlos also noted that he was going to try to resolve his current situation by learning to support and accept himself, rather than criticizing himself. He was going to work to be more positive in how he faced his choices so that he could truly choose a direction in life that seemed satisfying.

Again, in retrospect, I see how I could have taught a little more about the principles of Gestalt to Carlos, especially regarding the significance of what he could learn from this situation for how to be more effective in his life and in college, in particular. Specifically, I could have focused more on Carlos becoming more aware of how he was feeling self-support and lack of self-support in his body. I could do this in two ways: (1) have him focus on being more aware of his moment-to-moment feelings with respect to self-support and non-self-support, or (2) directly teach what I was seeing him experience in his work. While both are important, I truly feel that having Carlos become more aware of himself and his moment-to-moment feelings is the more important of the two because he then could be more present and aware "with his ongoing being," which I think is a big part of achieving completeness and effectiveness as a person.

Review of Initial GEC Work with Students

So, let's review what I was doing and learning in my initial Gestalt counseling work with students, as well as thoughts I was having about how to refine work with students so that they could better benefit from my introduction of Gestalt personal development principles. If we look at Sereta, we can see how her early experiences with a significant family member led her to develop an aspect of self that was non-supportive and mistrusting of experimenting regarding learning how to perceive and react to the world in different ways. Remember, also, that Sereta experienced this "lack of self-support learning" in great part in the physical posturing and emotions of her body. That is, Sereta learned to hold her body in certain ways to protect herself emotionally, which prevented her from experimenting with different behaviors in challenging situations.

If she were to try to be different, she would have to work through the habitual emotional body stances she had learned, which is what she did in her work with me, especially when she was in emotional upheaval. Sereta was learning to hold herself in a new way, to support her ability to change and be different and more effective in the world. I think the work with me helped Sereta to be more aware of how she was not supporting her growth. Also, Sereta's interaction and opening up to students led her to develop more self-support, physically and mentally, and forecasted a more positive and open attitude for how to face the psychological challenges important for achieving success in her physics course.

For Carmen and Carlos we see similar struggles and growth regarding how to develop greater self-support through improved self-awareness for how they had learned in their lives to not support their growth. Both learned in the present the value of trusting others - Carmen from her group members, and Carlos from a Latino counselor, in order to support their efforts at change and growth. Carmen learned in her body and mind that her interactions with her substitute parent had locked her into a way of being that was limited, a way that could only repeat the same non-effective efforts to challenges requiring personal change.

For Carmen, this self-position changed when she was able to stay with her hurt to the point of being able to look up and listen and see through her group members that there were options to the ineffective behaviors she had been using to handle her challenges. Carlos, too, after staying with the emotional pain of his self-rejecting, non-supporting self, learned that he was rejecting and not supporting his growth as a student and person. His owning of himself through use of "I" statements helped him see his internal war or split in his personality. He learned self-support when at the moment of intense pain and hurt he was supported by the loving, guiding hand of a Gestalt-trained Latino counselor.

At this point in my work with students, I was not satisfied that the students were receiving a clear and organized perspective for how Gestalt personal development principles could help them live more effective psychological lives. I wanted to create a Gestalt intervention that was more focused and impactful. I wanted students to leave my sessions with a clearer and more practical understanding for how the concepts of self-support, the Gestalt Cycle of Experience, and improved self-awareness could transform their efforts to live more effective, satisfying, and complete lives.

Reflecting on Persons of Color and Schooling: Classrooms of Shame and Seats of Doubt

There are, of course, other examples of where I as counselor worked with students and community members specifically addressing unfinished business related to school experiences. In one situation within a well-known drug reentry living facility, I was lecturing to a large group of ethnically diverse persons on how Gestalt counseling works to help one overcome fears and doubts that were developed in childhood. I had been provided instant credibility by a former resident and now resource person who said that I had served in his life as a substitute father because I had shared my genuineness and love toward him.

One of the persons in the audience was an African American woman of about forty-two years of age who said that she wanted to do some Gestalt work related to being more confident in school. During the work with this woman, she became tearful when she recounted her experiences in elementary school where she often "felt like I didn't belong." After a short discussion of this woman's experience, wherein it was evident that she held many strong and negative emotions related to her early school experiences, I arranged three chairs in a row, simulating a row of chairs in a classroom. I invited her to take a seat behind other members from the audience and to close her eyes and remember herself as a little girl in her classroom. The woman closed her eyes and immediately bent forward, grimacing slightly and began to show strong emotion. I asked her what she was experiencing and she replied that she felt a pain in her stomach. I then invited her to stay with her pain and to share what the pain was like. She said that the "pain was like an intense burning that wouldn't stop." When I asked her to speak in the present tense as if she was that pain, she bent forward more and whispered something that I could not hear. I softly touched the woman's shoulder and asked her to give more strength to this voice. The woman hesitated for a good minute, obviously struggling to allow her voice to come forward.

I again softly spoke to her, saying that I believed in her right to speak, and I supported her to give voice to what she was feeling. To this, she blurted out in a loud voice, "I can think! I can learn!" I asked the woman if she could see herself as a young person experiencing these feelings. She said she saw herself in the second grade, looking down and trying to hide from her teacher and the other students because she couldn't read well. I then asked the woman to speak to the child in a loving, supportive way and to tell the child that she was with her, loved her, believed in her, saw her as special, and knew that she could learn.

Immediately, I saw her body lift up and her eyes brighten, brighten with increased hope. Following a short pause, I supported the woman to share with the group what she had learned in this exercise. She shared how painful it had been for her experiencing the many, many hours that she spent in elementary school wanting to speak up about her belief in her ability to learn. She told the group and they, in turn, verbalized support for her that she could indeed go to college and use her mind to learn and to achieve success.

In another situation with a group of Latina women who were part of the University of California program called Puente, where I had introduced the participants to GEC, one of the women asked to work on her lack of confidence in her ability to learn to write English. Seeing obvious signs of tension in the woman, I asked her to describe how she felt whenever she thought about writing or actually sat down to write. The woman described feeling "scared and doubtful" that she was smart enough to learn to read and write English. I asked the woman to describe more in depth what she felt in her body when she thought about writing. The woman said that she felt a tension in her legs, as if she wanted to run away. I asked her if this reminded her of any situations in her early school experiences. With a surprised look, she answered "Yes!" and that she could remember a time when she was in an English class and she was very frightened that a substitute teacher would find out that she was "dumb and couldn't do English." The woman recounted the many times that she slipped out of the class before the teacher came in to avoid being "found out" by the teacher.

I therefore decided to arrange a classroom-like situation and role-play what the woman had experienced as a child in school. To this end, I had the group arrange chairs in rows and asked everyone to take a seat. The woman said that she didn't want to reexperience this part of her past. And to this, I said, "Maybe we'll do something different." Once the chairs were arranged in rows, I asked the woman to sit in the chair closest to the door. When she took a seat, I inquired after her feelings. She said that she felt "like running out the door." To this, I asked her to speak as if she was the door. Speaking as the door, the woman said, "I'm going to shut you in so everybody sees how dumb you are." When I then asked her how she felt as the door, the woman responded that she felt "mean and angry." At this point I thought about inquiring if she could connect this "mean and angry" experience to an earlier life experience with a significant other, but I decided on a different approach.

I shared with the group that I was going to experiment and play a supportive and caring teacher who wanted all the children to feel good about themselves as learners. I then requested all the women to pretend they were students in the class. I surveyed the room to determine whether anyone had any questions about learning English that they wanted to ask. All of them had questions. I asked all of the women present to pretend to be very inquisitive students who were really excited about learning English. Most of the women raised their hands with enthusiasm to role play, as if they were excited and had questions to ask about writing. The woman with the issue about writing seemed hesitant to participate. I therefore supported the woman to raise her hand and ask a question. The woman tentatively looked at her group companions, but finally raised her hand as if she had a question.

To this I called out her name and said with enthusiasm, "Let's see what question (the woman's name) has!" The woman hesitantly asked, "How do you use a comma?" To this question, I enthusiastically responded with, "What a great question!" and I then also asked the other would-be students, "to raise their hands if they saw this as a great question." All the students raised their hands and they chimed in that they felt the question was very good and that they also wanted to know how to use a comma.

I asked the woman who had asked the question if she knew some rules for using a comma. The woman looked around at her would-be classmates and hesitatingly said, "Yes, I think I do." As the would-be teacher, I answered with "Great. Let's hear what you have to say!" The woman then hesitantly shared a rule that she thought related to the use of commas, and I as the counselor/teacher with enthusiasm congratulated the woman on providing useful information to the class. At the same time, I asked the role-playing group members if they appreciated the ideas shared by their classmate. The group members in chorus said, "Oh yes, she's really great and helpful!"

At this point, the Latina with the concern about her writing became visibly emotional, and I then stepped closer to the woman and held her hand as she began to cry. This lasted for a couple of minutes, after which the woman shared how aware she had become through this role play about the level of hurt and shame that she had carried within herself, in her body, as a result of her early experiences in school. She vowed to the group that she "would make a serious effort to start believing in" her ability to learn to write well and that she would begin to work more seriously on developing her writing skills.

As a postscript to this group role play, a couple of other group participants shared that while taking part in the dramatization, they got in touch with some intense feelings related to shaming and demeaning experiences that they had experienced in their early schooling. One woman, in particular, mentioned how she had been filled with terror (can you imagine what as a little girl the experience of terror was like in her body?) about the possibility of going up to the front of the class to do work on the chalkboard. This led me to have the woman have a dialogue with the chalkboard, wherein the woman took the role of the chalkboard. The outcome of this work was that the woman became aware of how behind this fear of the chalkboard lay hurt feelings that she had long harbored toward a very close relative who had constantly criticized her as a young girl for not being as smart as her cousins.

So, what's happening in these latter anecdotes, and what was I learning about doing Gestalt work with persons of color? Clearly, childhood experiences, what I have earlier in this book called "Childhood Legacy," produce strong emotional binds of shame, doubt, and hurt that last and affect the adult personality. I was learning that doing Gestalt work could unloose these negative emotional binds to free a person to experiment with new ways of being as an adult, especially new ways of improving or changing long held and non-supportive emotions.

But, still, I struggled with the notion that a lot of what I was achieving was a result of my five years of training at the Gestalt Institute of San Francisco. I wanted to simplify my work to be able to teach some core principles of Gestalt personal development work to again offer a clear and practically useful introduction to how Gestalt personal development could be used by students to more effectively handle life's psychological challenges.

Chapter 8

2001: Transition to a One-session *Directive* GEC Session

The following testimonials are from two Latina (female) community college students and an eleventh-grade Latino (male) student following a forty-minute Gestalt Educational Counseling session with Dr. Rivas.

"Dr. Rivas, going back and forth on those chairs has been one of the most emotional experiences of my life. I was experiencing fear and emotional pain, and I was feeling lost. It was the most beautiful, scariest, painful, and relieving thing to have met myself for the first time. Thank you for that. The empty chair was a lot more helpful than a year in therapy." — Twenty-two-year-old *Latina Community College Student, Merritt College, Oakland, California.*

"Dr. Rivas, I experienced today something I never had experienced in my life, like I got rid of something I have been holding on for so long. Doing that empty chair thing was new for me, which helped me a lot because after all that I didn't have that bad feeling in my chest anymore." — Nineteen-year-old *Latina Community College Student, Merritt College, Oakland, California.*

"I felt like a big weight was lifted off my shoulders after doing the chair work. I breathed easier and I felt more confidence throughout my body." — Seventeen- year-old *Latino high school student, Oakland, California.*

The above three testimonials from students attest to the effect that one session of GEC can have with regard to supporting students' efforts to understand their psychological selves as well as begin to be more effective in their studies. Let's look at what I think these testimonials communicate regarding the personal growth experience of these students:

"Experiencing fear and emotional pain and feeling lost;" "meeting myself for the first time," and "getting rid of something I have been holding for a long time in my life;" "I felt like a big weight was lifted off my shoulders after doing the chair work; I breathed easier and I felt more confidence throughout my body."

Sadly, yet happily for both the students and myself (because I have learned that through Gestalt personal development work challenging personal, social, and educational issues can be successfully addressed), many students experience emotional challenges in their education that are tied to negative childhood emotional experiences, what I have called our "Childhood Legacy." These experiences create what Gestalt psychologists call "shame binds." Shame binds prevent individuals from experiencing an emotionally unified, balanced, and centered self in mind and body, and instead create lasting negative behavioral limitations that result in ineffective emotional habits that lessen the ability to complete experiences that call for emotional balancing, change of internalized behavioral habits, and possibilities for psychological growth.

This growth is needed to develop an integrated (unified) and effective personality. As I have shared in the counseling anecdotes in the previous chapter, over the last twenty-plus years, I have conducted Gestalt Educational Counseling with thousands of persons, individually and in groups, with a special focus on high school and college students of color who face unique challenges in and out of school. My conclusion is that many students' emotional challenges can be effectively addressed if negative childhood emotional legacies are first brought to awareness by teaching the principles of the Gestalt Cycle of Experience, and then by physically integrating the negative childhood emotional legacies (by doing Gestalt personal development work) into the present functioning of the person so as to facilitate growth into a more unified and effective functioning self. This is the essence of the more focused GEC approach that I have developed to "teach" the power of Gestalt personal development work for improved psychological functioning.

I now want to look more closely as to the why and how of GEC. The term "directive" in the title of this chapter relates to an approach to counseling with multicultural populations when the counselor directly introduces knowledge related to psychological growth and provides guidance options to the client for handling challenges, rather than relying on a non-directive approach where little direct guidance is given to persons for what choices might be more useful to them. The non-directive approach is the method often used in counseling and therapy, with the underlying rationale being to support an individual to develop his or her own psychological strength and choices for life direction. In an article entitled, "The Prescriptive Relationship in Academic Advising as an Appropriate Developmental Intervention with Multicultural Populations" (Brown and Rivas, 1994), my colleague Tom Brown and I argued, with supportive proof, that many students of color progress more effectively through advising and counseling if provided with more directive versus non-directive guidance. This is because lack of familiarity and understanding on the part of these populations with the methods and processes of advising and counseling very often limits the effectiveness of these interventions.

With a more directive approach rather than having to guess about what is happening in counseling, the counselor provides more direct advice about options available for psychological growth. Tom Brown and I also argued that directive advising and counseling is on a continuum where non-directive advising and counseling is indeed powerful, but is an end goal to be moved to rather than used before an individual is developmentally ready. I have incorporated a more directive approach into Gestalt Educational Counseling (GEC) so as to support a greater understanding of the methods and processes of Gestalt personal development work for persons who are not knowledgeable or familiar with counseling and therapy theory or practice. Also, my experience has been that a more directive counseling approach is more effective in supporting the increased confidence, learning, and understanding of multicultural populations for how Gestalt personal development ideas can improve their psychological effectiveness.

As I have shared, in my counseling with students both individually to support facing emotional difficulties in taking my psychology classes or with general study in college as well as in Gestalt group workshops at conferences and with academic leadership programs such as MESA, EOPS and Puente, I was feeling good about my effectiveness to help students become more psychologically effective in their lives by sharing Gestalt concepts and exposing them to Gestalt counseling work. Nevertheless, I saw my success as limited with respect to long-range impact on students because I felt I was not providing a well-organized learning experience with specific "take-aways." What I wanted for individual students and workshop participants was a straightforward and well-organized guide that they could then use on an ongoing basis to take responsibility and assume greater control of their life's emotional challenges. I wanted to develop a more simple and straightforward method to teach and introduce students, community members, and counseling practitioners to the power of Gestalt personal growth methods. I came up with a one-session Gestalt Educational Counseling (GEC-1) method to do this.

The One-Session Introduction to
Gestalt Educational Counseling (GEC-1)

The GEC-1 teaching and learning approach for applying Gestalt concepts to resolving one's psychological challenges involves the following five phases of knowledge sharing and actual Gestalt work:

Phase 1: An introduction to the importance of developing Gestalt-oriented awareness for how one is experiencing self in present psychological challenges, as well as how a person's present strategies are often self-limiting, ineffective emotional and behavioral habits resulting from negative childhood learning experiences (again, what I call our Childhood Legacy). To strengthen this introduction, I include personal sharing as to how I developed greater understanding of my ineffective emotional habits and developed psychological strength through Gestalt counseling work.

Phase 2: Sharing a personal anecdote from my life related to how I learned ineffective emotional habits during my childhood and review of the Gestalt Cycle of Experience as a model for becoming aware of how one can ineffectively experience emotional challenges, as well as how to grow and progress through emotional difficulties.

Phase 3: Doing empty chair work to bring persons face-to-face with how their current ways of reacting to emotional challenges are an outgrowth in many cases of individuals having been psychologically overwhelmed by difficult childhood emotional experiences when they didn't learn "self-support.".

Phase 4: Supporting persons to assume "adult-based" responsibility for handling the emotional challenges of their lives by consciously releasing their child-self from continuing to try to handle adult psychological challenges.

Phase 5: Review of how the person doing chair work has been affected by the work, which includes individual reflection or compassionate feedback from the counselor or group participants regarding how they experienced the person doing chair work, as well as how group participants may have been affected by observing the work. Again, I have used this approach with much success with community college students, high school students, community growth groups, and counseling training groups since 2001.

Phase 1: An introduction to Gestalt psychological growth concepts to connect persons' current ineffective ways of handling psychological challenges to negative ineffective habits developed as a result of difficult situations experienced in childhood.

The initial part of GEC-1 is a general introduction to Gestalt concepts to improve personal growth, which I've noted in Chapter 2. When I do Gestalt interventions with individuals or groups, I make this connection in a general way. First, by sharing my experience of having done Gestalt personal development work, sharing how I learned through challenging emotional experiences to become aware of how what I have called my "Childhood Legacy" impacted how I learned to handle my adult psychological challenges, e.g., how I emotionally responded initially with apprehension and doubt to having to teach to a large group of students a mandatory freshman orientation class where many of the students acted negatively toward me for having to be in the class.

I also share how Gestalt personal development work helped me to support myself to develop better psychological health in my life. Importantly, to make sure my messages are being understood, I consistently ask individuals or workshop participants for questions and feedback regarding how well I have communicated the usefulness of doing Gestalt personal development work.

Following my sharing of the positive impact that doing Gestalt work had on my personal development, I then do an awareness exercise to have persons experience the connection between present psychological functioning and ineffective psychological strategies developed as a result of difficult childhood experiences. To do this, I ask persons in individual sessions or all persons in large group sessions if they can get in touch with how they physically feel when they are frustrated by an inability to effectively face and manage a difficult emotional challenge in their present life. Once persons acknowledge their ability to get in touch with their bodily reactions, e.g., tight throat, headache, shaky legs, etc., I ask the individuals or group members to focus on those feelings and at the same time notice if they can see an image of themselves as a child having similar feelings.

In individual sessions, most persons are able to connect their present-day feelings of frustration to an image of themselves in a specific challenging situation in childhood where they were experiencing negative emotions. In large groups, many persons nod yes to acknowledge that they can connect their feelings related to present psychological challenges to a visual image related to a difficult childhood situation. With this exercise, I make an experiential connection between present and past, and go on to share how knowledge of the Gestalt Cycle of Experience can be used to re-do ineffective past emotional learning and develop more psychological strength to handle challenges in their present lives.

Phase 2: Introduction to the Gestalt Cycle of Experience and how knowledge and practice of progressing through the Cycle can improve psychological functioning.

Before doing any Gestalt work, I move into Phase 2 of GEC-1, an introduction and review of the Gestalt Cycle of Experience, which is a description of a step-by-step process where a person effectively experiences, resolves, and grows through a difficult psychological challenge. The Gestalt Cycle of Experience emphasizes a positive growth process where there is movement from getting in touch with sensations in one's body, as well as developing awareness for how one's "sense-making-self" ala, "coming to our senses," is an organismic response to an emotional challenge to "mobilizing or gathering one's physical energy" to recognize one's needs and wants and how they related to resolving a challenging psychological situation.

"Action" is the next step in the Cycle, where one acts to meet one's needs and wants. This is followed by "Contact" with one's developing self, wherein the whole self is moved by the positivity of one's actions in support of resolving a psychological challenge. This is then "assimilated" into the overall functioning of the person's personality. Another term I like to use for assimilation is integration, wherein a person integrates (re-organizes a more unified self) into a new, more complete self which is based on the ongoing resolution of life's psychological challenges. The final step in the Cycle is "Withdrawal" from the current situation, wherein a person moves on with life with a more "Complete Self," who is more adept at assuming responsibility (self-support) to handle future psychological challenges as new life challenges emerge (Gestalt "Emergencies"). When introducing the Gestalt Cycle of Experience, I address how one can get stuck in moving through the Cycle because of personal emotional blocks related to movement through steps in the Cycle, e.g., individuals may experience difficulty being in touch or aware of their feelings/senses or may have difficulty mobilizing energy to take action, etc. In my introduction to the Gestalt Cycle of Experience, I emphasize the importance of: (1) becoming aware of movement or lack of movement through the Cycle; and (2) the importance of developing "self-support" to experiment and adapt one's responses to challenges as one progresses through the Cycle.

Phase 3: Doing empty chair work to come face-to-face with the experience of how one's current way of reacting to emotional challenges can be connected to negative childhood emotional challenges.

GEC-1 Phase 3 involves doing chair work where participants act out a psychological drama with guidance from a trained Gestalt counselor, wherein the adult-self interacts with the "hurt child-self" in an imaginary role-play centering on a psychological challenge experienced in childhood. Importantly, prior to reviewing Phase 3, I talk about what may happen when individuals connect present-day feelings to difficult childhood experiences. For example, before I introduce this process, I review possible emotional reactions that can be experienced in movement through the Cycle, including surprise, confusion, anger, resentment, shame, etc. I also reinforce that this is the beginning of a process of personal development through self-awareness that can significantly improve a person's psychological growth and effectiveness.

In over twenty years of doing this work, I rarely witnessed (maybe twice, and I was able to address this with the individual) anyone being emotionally overwhelmed by this process. But remember, I constantly emphasize to persons that they, like me, can learn to get to know and become aware of their psychological self, including needs for growth and opportunities that present themselves for personal development. I also communicate that participation in GEC is voluntary, which has allowed many persons to slowly develop the strength and courage to participate and do their growth work, much like I did when in Dr. Grossman's Gestalt class at the University of Minnesota.

There's another important point I want to address related to doing Gestalt chair work. Fritz Perls, the developer of Gestalt therapy, emphasized the importance of doing what is known as experiential work (direct experience of emotions) rather than merely "talking about" one's past or present problems (what Perls called mind-f-ing). I have witnessed the effectiveness and power of this method over and over and over again. In short, people can talk incessantly about their past or present problems with little progress in changing themselves for the better. However, when one directly experiences emotions (e-motion is the body in motion) and learns to support self to move through the Gestalt Cycle of Experience (which emphasizes experiencing and staying with difficult emotions until actively attempting to resolve these emotions), a person grows and changes in mind and body to be able to support new ways of supporting self when experiencing difficult emotions. So, as recommended by Fritz Perls, I do little "talking about" past experiences, and, as I have said, I focus on guiding a person to actively experience and support themself as they move through the Gestalt Cycle of Experience.

Back to the shortened version or GEC-1. Recall that prior to asking a person to do chair work between their adult-self and their hurt child-self, I have shared a personal growth experience of mine doing chair work, as well as connected how my childhood negative emotional learning made it a challenge for me in my adult challenges to move through the Gestalt Cycle of Experience. I can see in my writing that I am being extra careful in how I introduce Gestalt work with persons. This is because I have learned that many people have doubts when asked to share and experience difficult emotional experiences, either from the past or present.

Nevertheless, I have learned that almost 100 percent of the time, persons are very resilient in challenging themselves to grow, especially if they are sufficiently oriented to what is being asked of them by a caring person who is willing to share his or her emotional challenges and movement to personal growth in life. I have also learned that young persons are even more open to GEC than older persons, and I attribute this to their youthful openness to life. My thought is that they haven't yet learned to guard themselves as much as have older adults and that they respond very positively to opportunities for personal growth, especially if the person working with them is genuine, honest, caring, and accepting, à la Carl Rogers' (1961), conditions necessary for counselors to develop an environment to support personal growth work.

Another "truth" I have learned is that my interventions are much more effective with diverse populations if my work and background is introduced by someone who is known to the group and has good standing with the group, e.g., the Director of BAWAR, in Oakland, who had formerly been a student of mine in an abnormal psychology class. So, in short, an important part of doing GEC, as with any other counseling approach, is to establish effective rapport with persons by showing caring and concern for the persons with whom one is helping.

Again, Phase 3 of GEC-1 is to do direct Gestalt work with persons using The Empty Chair Technique, specifically by acting out a drama where the adult-self, in role-play, interacts with the hurt child-self in a challenging childhood situation that has been identified by connecting present-day physical reactions to psychological challenges to similar feelings from a difficult childhood situation where a person's ability to understand and handle a challenge was overwhelming. The first question I pose is to the adult-self chair, and I ask how the adult-self feels when looking at the hurt child-self as they experience their difficult emotional situation. The feelings are always unique, but range from experiencing supportive feelings such as sadness, empathy, hurt, etc., to feelings of rejection, e.g., anger, disgust, to no feelings at all.

I then ask the person in the adult chair if there are words that accompany their feelings that they can share with their hurt child-self. Here, the response is almost 100 percent of the time an attempt to placate or calm or assure the child-self that they don't need to feel so bad in the situation and that "everything will be all right." My honest and caring response is that "things won't be alright," and, indeed, haven't been alright because the person is still having in their present life emotional reactions to situations similar to those they experienced in childhood!

At this point, my GEC-1 approach diverges from what I would call Gestalt therapy in which the therapist allows the chair work to continue more spontaneously and with little direct guidance from the counselor or therapist. In GEC-1, I have chosen to introduce Gestalt personal development work from a more directive perspective regarding how powerful this work can be to improve personal development. I therefore ask the person initiating this work if I can guide them through the chair work process to support them to become more aware of their emotional challenges, as well as how current emotional challenges may be connected to their Childhood Legacy of negative emotional learning, as well as to support them to resolve their challenges. Again, it is important that I previously have established rapport and trust with a person I am asking to do Gestalt personal development work because without such a bond I cannot guarantee a person's genuine involvement with the work and thus how effective the work will be.

After obtaining the participant's permission for me to guide the process of chair work, I then take persons through what I would call a loving, supportive experience regarding addressing and solving their childhood emotional challenges, all the while developing an awareness of difficulties in moving through the Gestalt Cycle of Experience. (This reminds me that I was often called "Dr. Love" in my many years of Gestalt group work because of the love and caring I constantly showed others.) The first step I use in this process is to have the adult-self say to the hurt child-self the following: "I see you in this difficult situation, and I want you to know that I feel everything you're feeling and thinking, and I am with you and support you totally as you go through this difficult emotional experience. I want you to know that I am with you, and that in fact, I *am* you!"

This is the beginning of what I consider a positive "reintegrative experience" where the adult-self is going to re-experience and reintegrate their hurtful childhood experience, but with support from the developed strengths of their adult-self as well as with the psychological strengths, guidance, and support of the Gestalt counselor. I also want to add that sometimes a person does not directly repeat my words, and in such instances, I retain their expressions because they come from their direct experience of the self. In fact, if a person doing chair work adds a word or phrase, this expression may signal a powerful need on the part of the person that may require extra attention and focused work.

An example of this might be that a person adds to "I am with you," by saying, "and I don't want you to doubt that I am with you!" This may signal many things, even a real doubt that the adult-self can truly interact with the hurt child-self. At times when I have heard added statements made by a person doing chair work beyond what I recommend, I might take a detour in the work and ask the person to get in touch with what they have brought up, e.g., possible doubts they might have about being genuine with their hurt child-self. Continuing, after the supportive sharing from the adult-self to the hurt child-self in the difficult emotional situation, I ask the participant to switch from the adult-self chair to the child-self chair.

The change from the adult-self chair to the hurt child-self chair is always very poignant, being a mixture of sadness and regret or optimism and positivity. Importantly, I watch for the person's bodily reactions to the change in chairs. These bodily reactions can range from taking a relieving breath, to tearing up and crying, to looking downcast and dejected. I then ask the person in the hurt child-self chair what they experienced regarding what the adult-self has shared about being totally in touch and supportive of the experience of the hurt child-self in their difficult situation. The verbal response, which may take some time to be expressed, is usually, "I don't feel like I'm alone; I feel like there is someone with me who understands me and supports me!" Here I want to discuss my understanding of this initial step of doing GEC-1 empty chair work.

One of the most powerful forces that I have seen at work when I do GEC-1 work can be seen at this initial stage of the chair work, especially as I have structured the intervention. There is almost always a very positive response by individuals when the person in the adult-self chair communicates understanding, caring, and identification with the self in the hurt child-self chair. The response is always readily apparent and very moving, and, again, produces a very positive reaction from the individual in the child-self chair such as strong crying or pensive acceptance. Very often, in fact, one of the perceptions from the person, both during and following chair work, is that they never had acknowledged this "being united with self" nor the feeling of "being understood by the self." Along with this verbal statement, the person in both chairs acknowledges a sense of release of tension in the chest, and very often this is accompanied with a massaging of the chest area by the person doing chair work.

The latter experiences become even more moving and impactful in the next phase of the chair work when the person resumes the adult-self position. At this point, after getting what usually is a very emotionally positive response from the individual in the adult-self chair to having witnessed the response by the person in the hurt child-self chair to the initial statement of identification and support by the adult-self, I ask the person in the adult-self chair if he or she would be willing to say to the hurt child-self chair the following: "Along with what I have just said to you, I want you to know that without question to me you are wonderful and special, and that I love you completely and with my whole self!"

This request is very often accompanied with a very strong emotional response by both or one of the two selves. The emotions are powerful in their expression and usually involve, again, either strong crying or quiet, yet intense reflection. As with the initial statement of understanding and identification of the hurt child-self by the adult-self, this statement of love and recognition by the adult-self to the hurt child-self is met with a readily visible and intense level of emotional positivity, and what I can only call "feeling loved by a very, very important person in one's life – the self!" In fact, often individuals have openly acknowledged that they have never shown love to themselves!

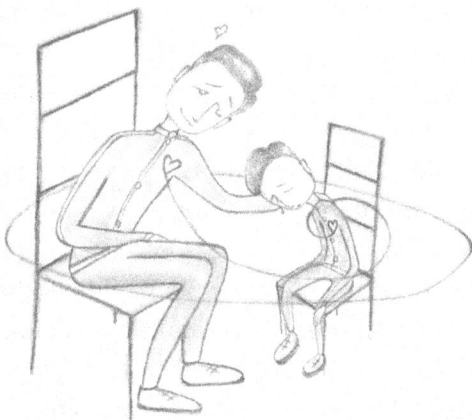

Adult-self to hurt child-self: "I want you to know that without question, to me you are absolutely wonderful, and that I love you completely and with my whole self!

There are two points I want to make related to the chair work I am describing. First, this work is not a simple movement from chair to chair with rote-like statements. Rather than rote acting out of phrases, the importance of the chair work is the recognition and acknowledgement by the counselor with the acknowledgement by the participant as to the shifting emotions and bodily reactions experienced by the person in the adult-self and child-self chairs. By way of example, I may ask a person to stop and feel the reaction to what is occurring in the chair work, or I may ask a person to repeat a statement that is being made if the restating of a phrase can add power to the ongoing interaction. I remember Dr. Abe Levitsky saying to me at different times during our counseling sessions, "It may be worthwhile for you to say the statement again that you just made, and take the time to experience in a more in-depth way what you are communicating to yourself and what you are feeling."

(Thank you again, Abe, for the love and caring that you often showed me!). Again, this work is very passionate, and I support the person to feel as in-depth as possible what they are experiencing

The second point related to GEC-1 chair work is that I can add, as I feel necessary, some diversion from the core GEC-1 work. This may be for reasons unique to the work of a particular person. One example of this is that at times some persons are not ready to make statements like, "I'm with you," or "I truly love you!" In fact, I have at times, though rarely, had persons say, "I hate you" or "I reject you" from the adult-self chair to the hurt child-self chair. In such instances, I accept what the person says and simply continue the chair work from that point by then asking the person to take the role of the hurt child-self, and to communicate their feeling and experience of the negative statements heard. And, as is generally the case, even though the adult-self may make a negative statement, the person, when assuming the hurt child-self chair, feels some positivity because they have heard the true feelings of the adult-self. To me this shows the importance of the experiencing of truth and honesty in how one expresses self in the process of doing personal development work.

Along with this perspective, the person in the hurt child-self chair often responds positively even though they have heard a negative statement aimed at them, adding, "At least he/she is communicating to me!" The main point is that I respect the person's honest expression from either chair position. In the end, however, I always move back to having the person expressing and experiencing love and acceptance from either chair, even though in some cases this may take a longer time to truly express. Related to this, Gestalt therapists talk about "fake it until you make it," wherein a person doing Gestalt work may have to pretend they feel and want to make positive statements to either their child-self or adult-self. This is called "experimentation," wherein a person experiments with different options of behaving or feeling.

Importantly, I have almost always witnessed that persons change from negative to positive feelings by pretending or doing experiments for the opposite of what they are feeling or experiencing. An example of this can be seen in my sharing of the angry VP work in Chapter 3 where Morgan Goodlander asked me to pretend to be a loving VP, opposite to the reality I experienced. This experiment led me to experience my need to truly feel in my body and mind my whole self, being loved, accepted, acknowledged, and respected as special by an authority figure in my life, who, in the end, represented receiving and integrating love from an authority figure similar to a father, which I don't recall experiencing as a child.

So, where have we arrived at in review of my practice using the shortened one-session version of GEC? In short, as I have structured GEC-1, I want the child-self to experience understanding, connection, and acknowledgement of "self being with the self" — "I am with you!" This connection for me reintegrates the childhood experience with a new perspective, that of not being alone, and being understood and supported. I have also structured the GEC-1 session to have the adult-self and hurt child-self experience love for the self, both giving and receiving. This experience is often a new and powerful experience, and when integrated into the self, including body and mind, becomes a powerful feeling of self-loving with which the individual can rely on and take into his or her future psychological challenges.

Phase 4: Supporting persons to assume "adult-based" responsibility for handling the emotional challenges of their life by consciously releasing their hurt child-self from continuing to try to handle the adult's psychological challenges.

The next phase of GEC-1, Phase 4, is to support the person to free the hurt child-self, which is a memory, to simply be a child, and not be responsible for addressing one's adult emotional challenges, and, at the same time, to have the adult-self assume responsibility for using their adult strengths, including their knowledge of the Gestalt Cycle of Experience and the Gestalt concept of "self-support" to face future emotional challenges. This phase is very important, and, as with all the other interventions, is an adaptation of a Gestalt intervention that I have experienced. The intent is to begin the separation of the hurt child-self from the daily life of the adult-self.

The way that I achieve support for letting go of the hurt child-self is to ask the person in the adult-self chair if they can recall any childhood activity that really made them happy, e.g., playing games with friends, drawing, reading, etc. While there have been a few instances where an individual does not recall such a time, the majority of persons readily respond to this question with a big smile and then are able to clearly describe the situation. To add power to this recollection, I ask for a description of what the child in the image is wearing, including the color of the clothing, as well as how the child is feeling. Individuals usually beam with joy as they see an image of themselves doing a favorite childhood activity. I then have the persons focus on this feeling of watching the beauty, peace, and joy of themselves doing an activity that brought them happiness in childhood. I also ask the person to say the following to the child-self in the happy situation:

"I see you being happy (in the situation), and I want you to know that I want you to live the rest of my life having fun in this special situation, and I want you to know that you don't have to try and help me anymore to handle my emotional challenges. I will take the responsibility of handling my life."

I follow this up by asking the person in the adult-self chair if the child-self is welcoming of simply living out life being happy (a new memory). If the child-self accepts, I move on. If the child-self hesitates or does not accept, which does occur occasionally, I have the person in the child-self chair express their concern, and I may spend a little time having both selves address and experience the doubt. As with most hesitation to move forward or express self-support, the experience of acknowledging true thoughts and feelings always proves useful in helping a person integrate the lack of connection or agreement between the perspectives of the person's experience in each chair.

A postscript to Phase 4 work is that I add a caveat to the act of creating separation between the child-self and the adult-self. Specifically, I have found with my own Gestalt work as well as in discussion with persons who have completed this work that sometimes the child-self, which is a cognitive memory which includes physiological reactions, does reinsert itself into the present life of the person even after stating that the adult-self will no longer use the hurt child-self to try to handle present-day challenges. What I do and what I recommend to others when they again get in touch with the hurt child-self when facing a current emotional challenge is to do a quick bit of work with the hurt child-self to support the separation of the two selves and to allow the adult-self to continue developing the self-support to be more effective in handling life's emotional challenges. I offer the following as an example.

When I was hired as Vice President of Student Services at Vista College in Berkeley, many of the counselors I directly supervised and with whom my office was in close physical proximity, were negative about my true commitment to being a VPSS rather than just using this position as a stepping stone to a college president position. As a reaction to their doubt and negativity toward me, I experienced a good amount of anxiety. When going to work one morning, I checked with my child-self to see whether he was playing or whether he was fretting about my current emotional challenge. I imagined him hiding behind my legs and saying, "I don't want to go there!" I decided to do an experiment with my child-self. I breathed and asked him to get on my shoulders and simply enjoy being a little boy on my shoulders, and that I would use my adult-self to handle my challenges at work. He agreed, and I went through my day being more calm, collected, and effective in my work. My child-self was happy during the day.

Phase 5: Review of how the chair work participant has been affected by the work, which includes individual reflection or compassionate feedback from the counselor or group participants regarding how they experienced the person doing chair work, as well as how they may personally have been affected by observing the work.

We have arrived at Phase 5, reflection on chair work by the client and supportive feedback from counselor or others if the work was done in a group setting. This phase is very important in that I see opportunity for participants to further clarify and integrate how the work may fit into their psychological approach to life. First, with individuals who have worked in groups, I ask that they choose different persons in the group and make the following statement: "(Group member's name), I want you to know that I am going to assume responsibility for my life, and not use my hurt child-self to try and resolve my emotional difficulties." Remember, again, this is a strategy that I learned in my Gestalt training as a member in group sessions.

Before the group member responds, I make a request that the person not give advice about how to handle problems; rather, I ask group members to share what they felt and experienced during a person's chair work. Responses from group members are varied; however, generally, the two most common responses over twenty years of my doing this work have been the following:

"I too experienced a similar emotional challenge as you during my childhood, and while you worked, I felt directly within me the impact with respect to my childhood emotional challenge. Also, I felt the power and benefit of you doing your work."

"I want to thank you for your courage in volunteering to do Gestalt chair work, and I hope to have the courage to do the same."

"I felt a lot of caring toward you and the emotional challenges you experienced. Thank you."

This reflection is a time when experienced emotions can be further felt and integrated by the person having done chair work as well as the person(s) giving feedback. For example, a person giving feedback may start to cry as he or she may recall some childhood emotional difficulty. I allow this, and often give time for the person crying to stay with their feelings. At the same time, I thank them for their honest feedback, and welcome them to doing Gestalt chair work in a future group meeting.

The last part of Phase 5 is an exercise where I ask persons to write down reflections of their experience. Again, this is to allow more thorough integration of the experience. The following is the assignment I give participants:

(1) Write down what you felt during the chair work as you moved back and forth in the chairs, paying special attention to how your body responded to the chair work; (2) Write down what you learned during the chair work.

Here I advise persons to open up to all the possible learning that was experienced, including new ways to hold one's body during difficult emotional situations, thoughts about self that were experienced, the experiences of new types of awareness, etc.

(2) Write down how you will use the learning from this experience in your future.

Participants' responses to these questions help me remember the participants' work, and helps the participants further integrate the work into their awareness of themselves and how they have handled emotional challenges in the past, as well as how they may need to change with respect to handling future emotional difficulties.

Summarizing the five phases of the GEC-1 approach, I want to emphasize that personal growth takes some considerable work. However, the work can be made more "agreeable," if you will, when it is approached from a positive "I can" perspective where the person doing GEC believes that the work will not be overwhelming, and that in the end, the work will prove very beneficial for the participant. This requires a considerable amount of competence and caring on the part of the counselor/practitioner that can be readily observed by GEC participants.

Being effective also requires that the counselor be committed to truly focusing on the experience and challenges being experienced by GEC participants. I think that I have progressed a long way (in my professional development) in offering an experience to persons whereby they learn an organized approach to supporting their personal growth, one where they can take away specific knowledge and skills to use in meeting emotional challenges in their lives. This was my intent, and I can breathe deeply in accepting this fact, as well as breathe peacefully that I have supported my values of helping diverse populations, including *"mi comunidad,"* to have a better understanding of psychology and Gestalt personal development concepts and strategies, in particular.

Chapter 9

Understanding the Gestalt Mantra "It is Our Birthright to Achieve Completeness": Readings

First, I want to give you a prelude to this chapter. I do this because when initially writing this chapter, I noticed that there was a lot of information. Immediately, I thought that this was too much information, but upon reflection, I concluded that the information, though extensive, is very important to the coming together of the focus of this book, namely, what does it mean for a person to achieve completeness; put another way, how do we develop a greater unity and wholeness as persons? I ask you to be patient with the number of ideas and authors that I present. Read slowly and focus your attention, because I have spent many, many hours poring over the books and authors I share with you. As such, I have abstracted what I consider essential for understanding the idea of developing a unified and complete self, and I hope that your careful reading will help you develop more clarity about your journey to completeness.

On August 19, 2023, I turned seventy-six. Think of it, 76. Wow! So, where am I in completing myself? And do I really understand what becoming complete means? Hmm, let me see. At this point, achieving completeness definitely means something different than I can recall from different times of my life — my childhood, adolescence, and now, adulthood. Reflecting on my past, I see that early on I was in great part focused on having a secure and happy place in the world with my family, then friends, family again, and then career. Nevertheless, there was more from life that I wanted, including a sense of peace and completeness within myself.

I have sought completeness in different ways: pleasures of the senses (sex, alcohol, sports diversions, joy with family and friends); development as a professional (seeking more responsibility, creativity, and advancement); and psychological and spiritual growth. With regard to the latter, I was raised Catholic, but different experiences made me turn away from the Catholic religion. I tried alternative religions, including the Unitarian and Bahia faiths, but to no avail. I looked a bit at Buddhist philosophy, but did not then find answers that I sought with respect to understanding something about myself beyond what I was already doing in my day-to-day life.

I was at peace at a certain level, but I sought more. What, you may ask? I would say that I was searching for being more complete as a person; however, completeness was more of a feeling and not a clear concept nor a clear goal for me. I had to learn more. I have shared that in talks, group work, and counseling sessions, I often lead with the Gestalt quote, "It is our birthright to achieve completeness," and that when I asked how many persons want to achieve completeness, everyone have always raised their hands — yes, everyone! I'm always amazed by the rapidity and totality of peoples' affirmation that they want to achieve completeness. But I wondered what does completeness mean to all those that eagerly raise their hands?

Another quote I like to share with audiences is, "Percept without concept is blind," that is, we must understand the conceptual meaning of what we perceive and think about, or indeed, we might be blind to the true essence of an idea such as the meaning of becoming complete as a person. Therefore, in this chapter I want to look at what "achieving completeness" means from a conceptual perspective and then from the perspective of wise "seekers" who have spent their careers studying and writing books which attempt to understand the human personality. I am certain that each author holds part of the key to opening the door of what it means to be complete as a person. And, for my part, I will at the same time continue elaborating on what achieving completeness has meant to me in my life.

Beginning to Make Meaning of
"Our Birthright to Achieve Completeness"

First and foremost, what do the words in this quote mean, and especially, the word completeness? From a dictionary definition, completeness as an noun means: "(1) having all the necessary or appropriate parts; and (2) [often used for emphasis] to the greatest extent or degree; total." As a verb, completeness means: "(1) finish making or doing; or (2) make [something] whole or perfect."

So, completeness is defined as a quality we can have or an action we can undertake and complete. A question that comes to mind is, "What are the parts or aspects of ourselves that make us complete? The word "appropriate parts" is interesting because it points to what in ourselves is most relevant for our being complete as persons. In this regard, I am reminded of the words of Nathaniel Branden in "The Six Pillars of Self Esteem." "Self-esteem, *fully realized* (I have added italics as being analogous to completeness), is the experience that we are appropriate to life and to the requirements of life." A question related to being complete would be, "What makes us appropriate to life?" Another term of interest in the definition of completeness is, "to the greatest extent or degree." This is important because it points to a potential degree or level of completing oneself that we can achieve: How much and in what ways can we complete ourselves as human beings?

Questions, questions, questions; but let's continue our search for the meaning of completeness. To me the phrase, "It is our birthright to achieve completeness," refers to an undertaking commonly shared by all of us and begun at birth, signaling that becoming complete is a natural right of being human. So, what is this right? I go back to a drama that I often act out when I give talks: I get down on all fours, and I show how we slowly progress from being on hands and knees to standing upright. While dramatizing a process that goes back and forth between moving forward and falling down with seeming lack of progress, a child does not give up, does not say negative things about her or himself, but continues, goes on and on, to *complete* the act of standing and walking.

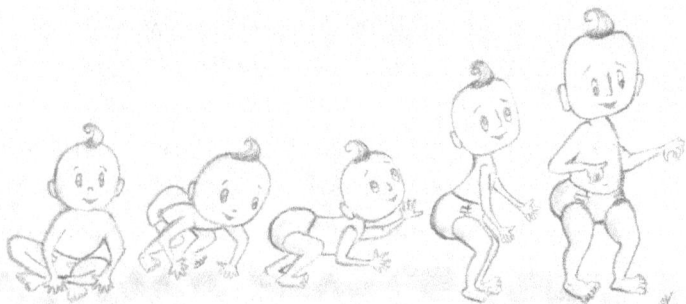

...A child does not give up, does not say negative things about her or himself, but continues, goes on and on, to *complete* the act of standing and walking.

As humans, we have spent thousands of years evolving to a point when we stand upright and can move through the world to find our way as unique persons. For me, here lies what is at the core of what it means "to achieve completeness." Each of us goes about defining our individual way of being — who we are, and how we want to be in the world. In fact, this is a right that humanistic psychologists say with which we are born. "Each individual has great freedom in directing his or her future, a large capacity for personal growth, a considerable amount of intrinsic worth, and an enormous potential for self-fulfillment." (Plotnik and Kouyoumdjian, 2011.)

Robert Kegan, in his book the "Evolving Self," writes that humans are "meaning-makers," that is, we construct our reality by actively building the meaning of our life experiences. I like this perspective because it argues that each of us has the ability to define who we are by using our mind to understand what our existence means to us, as well as how we want to go about organizing or completing our understanding of our self and how we want to express our self in the world. Much like the drive to stand and learn to walk, I believe that we also have a drive to use our mind to progressively clarify who we are as individuals, to "know the truth about ourselves!"

Gestalt perceptual psychology (the field of psychology that studies human perception) puts forth that our brain has seven operating principles or laws that help us organize our experiences in the world: figure-ground, proximity, closure, continuity, symmetry, similarity, and simplicity. These rules or processes are at work in our brains as we perceive and make sense of ourselves through our life experiences. It is through these processes that we see and define our self-concept. Completeness must surely involve having a clear mind so as to define what is right and wrong for the experience of our self as we progress through life.

So, my conclusion is that defining who we are, our self-concept, is a major part of what "becoming complete" means. With regard to perception, Gestalt therapy refers to the concepts of figure-ground and closure as major forces that guide movement through what Gestalt therapists call the Gestalt Cycle of Experience, which I see as a process that underlies our move to becoming complete as persons. We, in fact, individually perceive and give meaning to the world in order to complete what we determine to be important for us. For example, going through the Gestalt Cycle of Experience, we are organizing into the definition of our self-concept what stands out in our day-to-day lives (Figure versus Ground), and what is important in the ongoing process of completing self (Closure). I personally have seen myself over and over organize and reorganize who "Mario" is and how I want to express "I".

What is figure versus ground in my self-perception continuously has changed because of my drive to face and make sense of the realities or truth of my life. I have continuously sought closure in my day-to-day experience of myself, all aimed to achieve greater clarity regarding who I am as an individual. In childhood, I watched myself within my *"familia,"* experiencing love from my *mama y mi hermano,* and fear, anger, and shame from my papa. I recall being confused by what I too often remember as an unorganized chaos due to the inconsistency and insecurity that existed in my early family life. But I had few words for this at that time.

Nevertheless, my brain was helping me organize and make meaning of my experiences. Recall the cartoon image of chaos that first stood out for me (figure-ground) as an adult when I struggled to see and organize undefined and chaotic emotions in my life, emotions that were related to my initial childhood perceptions of my family experience. What I remembered were vague pictures and related bodily sensations from my childhood experiences because there were no clear words that I could use to remember my past. This greater awareness of myself I had to build. As a person, I was being moved forward toward completing my unique self!

Through all the difficult times of my childhood, I can say that I was constantly searching for completing "Little Mario" — "*Mayito*" as I was known to my mama and brother. I clearly remember the goodness and clarity of what it means for me to have a good life — to have love, understanding, and support from others around me. For me, it was the love of my mother and brother. Again, I think that throughout my childhood experiences, I was seeking closure and a sense of connectedness and continuity in my life experiences. Within the love of my *mama and hermano*, I slowly but progressively learned to define myself with more and more clarity, and to act in ways that supported the authoring and completing of my "unique self," a self which wanted, needed, and valued the experience of having a complete family.

Before moving on, I want to look further at the writing of Robert Kegan in "The Evolving Self" (2009) and the idea of completeness as a verb or action. Kegan writes:

"The subject of . . . The Evolving Self . . . is the person, where "person" is understood to refer as much to an activity as to a thing — an ever-progressive motion engaged in giving itself a new form . . . the Evolving Self . . . is about human being as an activity. It is not about the doing that a human being does; it is about the doing which a human being is (pages 7-8)."

"The doing which a human being is" is an important phrase for this chapter in that it argues that who we are is how we act, and, by extension, how we organize the meaning of our actions (meaning-making) into the authoring of our unique self. William James, considered to be the father of psychology in the United States, is quoted as having said, "To be is to do." And, so, we arrive at the Gestalt Cycle of Experience as a "doing" of who we are (Sensation, Awareness, Mobilization of Energy, Action, Contact, Assimilation, Withdrawal). Importantly, the emphasis is on the activity of being human, and so I contend that to complete self is indeed an ongoing process or activity of giving ourselves a new form!

Books, Books and More Books as
I Have Searched for Completeness

I now want to turn to my long-time search for the meaning of completeness as this plays out in the act of reading books. This morning I was contemplating why I have read so many psychology-related books. My love of books did not result from reading at home as a child, because my mama was working long hours cleaning houses and did not have the time to help me read, and she did not speak much English. Rather, my love of reading started in high school when I watched with interest some students who always had a book in their hand. Their focused reading inspired me and communicated to me that books meant something. But, what?

My growing interest in books continued indirectly when as a teenager I hung around Telegraph Avenue at the fringes of the University of California Berkeley campus, and as I sometimes walked through the many bookstores looking at interesting titles. When I finally returned to college after initially failing at Laney College, I began focusing on psychology books because I was majoring in psychology. I remember that I would regularly go to the bookstores on Telegraph Avenue to search out books by such psychologists as Abraham Maslow, Karen Horney, Harry Stack Sullivan, Eric Fromm, Sigmund Freud, etc., that could take me further into the theories and ideas to which I was being exposed in my college courses.

While university undergraduate libraries such as the Tolman Hall Undergraduate Psychology Library at UC Berkeley were great places to look for a book, there was something different and better that I felt when I could pick out a title in a bookstore and hold the book in my hand and possibly own it. I think I felt the power in my body and mind related to how these authors could help me find out who I was and how I could achieve the best and most complete Mario.

And this power was not solely in my mind, but translated to my daily life. I recall one day when I was experiencing a great deal of anxiety, and, with my twin one-and-a-half-year-old daughters Elena and Tita, I went searching for books to help me understand what I was experiencing, and, possibly, how to improve the anxiety I was feeling. I remember picking up a book titled, "If You Meet the Buddha on the Road, Kill Him" by Sheldon Kopp. When I opened the book and read the introductory paragraphs, I recall experiencing a calm wash over my anxiety from Kopp's recounting of an anecdote from his therapy work with clients. He wrote that persons came to him almost as if needing someone to carry them, to hold them in their doubts and fears about life.

This, indeed, is what I felt as I looked for help. Kopp wrote that instead of responding to an individual's need to be held, he would metaphorically step aside and let them fall and would add, "I won't carry you, but I'll walk alongside you as you search for the strength and meaning of your life!" From this reading of a single paragraph, I went from doubt and insecurity and was back to learning how to stand and walk as a complete person! At present, I can feel in my hands as I type, the peace and hope I felt immediately as I turned the pages of Kopp's inspiring book. Truly, books have been a major part of the goodness and completeness of my life.

So, what have I learned from my readings about achieving completeness as a person? Let me share key ideas related to achieving completeness from psychology-related books that have inspired me to clarify who I am and what I want from life, as well as share ideas from personal growth books that have significantly helped me be more effective at being and completing who I am. In the end, I will connect the ideas from these special authors to books on Gestalt theory and practice to show how my journey to personal and professional development has led me to focus on using Gestalt personal growth ideas and methods to help myself and others improve psychological growth and the move to personal completeness. I will also share in my next chapter a practical method I have developed, "The 0-100% Competence Method and Circle of Development" that I use when helping others organize their search for meaning and completeness. It is my hope that you will read some or all of the books I talk about to find answers relevant to your personal self-awareness pursuits.

What and how we think, feel, and act lead to our self-esteem: *Saber, Entender, Sentir, Escoger y Hacer*. I came up with this phrase in Spanish to communicate a process of living that aims toward our being complete. We can think and know (*Saber y Entender*) and not feel anything; but adding the power of feeling (*Sentir*) to the first two actions means that if we connect what we think about to what we experience in our body we can then be more integrated as a person and ready to choose a life direction and act with clarity and commitment (*Escoger y Hacer*). Choosing and taking action to fulfill one's values, wants, and desires completes the process of acting as oneself in a clear and unified manner.

In this regard, Nathaniel Branden's books on self-esteem have helped me understand how thinking, feeling, and acting affect how I feel about how we see ourselves — our self-esteem. "Self-esteem is the ability to think and cope with the challenges of life. Self-esteem is the feeling of being worthy, deserving, and entitled to assert one's needs and wants, to achieve one's values, and to enjoy the fruits of one's efforts." Branden offers this definition of self-esteem in his book "The Six Pillars of Self Esteem." Branden's "pillars" are a metaphor for the strengths that provide essential support for a person to fully develop and act on his or her potential to be a complete person.

Both the pillars' book and one of Branden's original works, "The Psychology of Self Esteem," had a major impact on my development, both as a person and professional psychologist. Both very readable books, Branden's writing immediately appealed to me because of his insistence that individuals must use their mind to clarify who they are and then to live by standing erect, both within themselves as well as with others, to speak and act "their truth" about what they think and what they believe to be correct for

themselves in the world (The Pillars of "Living Purposefully" and "Self-Assertiveness"). My conclusion from reading Branden's works is that our expression and achievement
of self-esteem is one of the main cornerstones for achieving
completeness, especially because it supports the actions of
our "real self."

Nathaniel Brandon's six pillars of self-esteem are the following:

1. The practice of living consciously;
2. The practice of self-acceptance;
3. The practice of self-responsibility;
4. The practice of self-assertiveness;
5. The practice of living purposefully;
6. The practice of personal integrity.

The strength of what these pillars communicate is that
they are grounded in two basic qualities of being that support the development of self-esteem: Self-efficacy and self-
respect. Branden defines self-efficacy as "confidence in our
ability to learn and do what we need to do in order to
achieve our goals." He adds, "Self-efficacy is not the conviction that we can never make an error. It is the conviction that
we are able to think, to judge, to know — and to correct our
errors. It is trust in our mental processes and abilities." The
emphasis on trusting our mind, which all of us inherit at
birth, is to work toward clarifying what we want to know,
defining who we are, and, finally, expressing who we are!
Self-respect, the other basis for our self-esteem, is the act of
feeling the worth or value of ourselves, which we support
when we express and act out our individual needs and
wants. The feeling of worth is evident in Branden's six

pillars, because when we value and accept our self, we have the internal strength to support our actions to complete our self.

One of the values of Branden's pillars book is that he devotes a chapter to each of the six pillars of self-esteem, and provides ideas and exercises to clarify how each of the pillars can help us develop more self-esteem. For example, some suggestions for how we can live more consciously are the following: Being receptive to new knowledge and willing to reexamine old assumptions; being willing to see and correct mistakes; seeking always to expand awareness — a commitment to learning — therefore a commitment to growth as a way of life.

Branden also explains how awareness of our biology can help us live more consciously. He shares that Wilhelm Reich ("Character Analysis") defined a biological-psychological process whereby our negative emotional experiences build up in us a "body armor," and that this body armor prevents clarity of thought and action because it blocks our energy to think and act freely. If we work on releasing this body armor, such as by doing "Rolfing," a form of intense body massage that releases pent up emotions, or, for me, doing Gestalt work, we can live more consciously because our bodies are freed up to bridge the connection between knowing and understanding to feeling, and then to choosing and acting with supportive and clarifying feelings (*Saber, Entender, Sentir, Escoger y Hacer*): Our life energy to act out and complete our uniqueness then flows more freely through our body!

Also, in each of the pillar chapters, Branden provides us with sentence completion activities to help us live more consciously. The following are just a few of the sentence stems offered by Branden: Living consciously to me means "If I bring 5 percent more awareness to my activities today…; If I bring 5 percent more awareness to how I deal with people today…; If I bring 5 percent more awareness to my most important relationships…; When I reflect on what on what happens when I bring 5 percent more awareness to each of the latter, what happens… Some other powerful sentence stems are: "If I bring 5 percent more awareness to my insecurities…; If I bring 5 percent more awareness to my depression…"

These sentence stems have helped me develop more awareness and conscientiousness about important aspects of my day-to-day life, and have helped me clarify what choices are open to me to raise my self-esteem. As Branden notes, also at the core of our self-esteem is our freedom to make choices. I conclude that when we make choices that support acting on our individual uniqueness, we support our self-efficacy and self-respect!

I want to add a couple of thoughts of mine related to Branden's six pillars. First, I share a good deal of Branden's ideas because I want you to be introduced to his work in a thorough manner so that this might lead you to pick up his books to see if they can be helpful in your effort to grow psychologically and achieve completeness as a person. However, I want to add that while I see Branden's six pillars as powerful, I think they fall short in not acknowledging the essential nature of our shared humanity with others. As such, I would add a seventh pillar: The practice of respecting and supporting the development of all people around us.

Related to the latter point, Hanson and Medius in their book "Buddha's Brain: The Practical Neuroscience of

Happiness, Love, and Wisdom," hypothesize that building community may be the highest level of development in support of continued human evolution. So, to me, being complete is not solely an individual process; but, also, a community endeavor that in the act of sharing and supporting the growth of others helps each of us to achieve more individual completeness!

I have already introduced Robert Kegan's book "The Evolving Self," especially his idea that we are all "meaning-makers" and that what we do with meaning is to organize and author a self. I want to add more ideas of Kegan as they relate to the process of our authoring a self and working to become complete as human beings. Kegan notes that "meaning-making" is an evolutionary activity. By this I think he means that as human beings we have evolved by progressively clarifying with our minds and consciousness our uniqueness as human beings. In our present point of evolution as a species, Kegan defines this process as an ongoing activity of defining our separateness from the environment, including people and the physical world.

The actual process is that of "differentiation and integration," where we progressively define our difference from the world and then integrate that difference as an ongoing activity of authoring our personality or identify, which includes interdependence with the physical and social world. The "action" of this process involves Jean Piaget's concepts of "assimilation and accommodation," wherein we constantly take in information about the world (assimilation) and then integrate that information (accommodation) in a continuous and progressive manner to add new information for how we define or perceive our self.

Kegan says that this ongoing definition of the self goes

through different stages, with specific "psychobiologic transformations." The psychological transformations are our mental understanding of self and the biological transformation is the emotional (body-in-motion) experiences that accompany our changing perceptions of our self in distinction from others. According to Kegan, there are five stages or "balances" that define our clarification of self. These go from first being in the womb and the initial state of infancy, the *Incorporative Balance*, wherein we do not differentiate our individuality but are "embedded" in the world, at first as part of the womb and, then, in the initial months of life, as part of a nameless and formless environment.

Slowly, we experience our self, first by becoming more and more aware of our reflexes, the *Impulsive Balance*, wherein we begin to "grasp" the world, and then through perceiving our difference from others, the *Imperial Balance*, to then seeing ourselves as needing to interact with others to feel safety and esteem in the world, the *Interpersonal Balance*, and, finally, to experiencing how we are in an interdependent relationship with others as we share the energy of our world and universe, the *Interindividual Balance*. The term balance is important because Kegan emphasizes that in each stage of psychological development we achieve a new balance regarding our experience of our "self." With each new balance we perceive the world in a more complete way. Becoming complete, then, is an on-going activity wherein we define both our separateness and connectedness with the social and physical world around us, a process that continually develops more balance in our ability to act who we are.

In his book "Immunity to Change," Kegan introduces us to how our "progressive motion of giving ourselves a new form" can be blocked by emotions and related subconscious beliefs that we internalize as defense mechanisms from our early childhood experiences. In short, individual development and change toward more clarity of perceiving and acting our unique self is not an automatic process. This process can be blocked as a result of negative interaction with others.

Specifically, in the interpersonal stage of our development we can become over-dependent on the approval of others, and we can learn to turn away from defining ourselves as a unique person with a unique self-concept, and, instead, orient more toward fitting in or pleasing others. i.e. becoming a copy. In my Latin@ culture, for example, being part of the family is a very, very important value, so much so that many of us learn to think that who we are is defined solely by the family of which we are a part. The end result too often is that the family can define how we should be, and, because in childhood our family is profoundly important to our existence, we often give up following an equally important personal path related to our evolving self, the individual self.

Emotions are a key part of the process of our "evolving self" according to Kegan, wherein we often learn at a very deep level of our being to be afraid of acting different from how we have been socially conditioned. Kegan's "immunity to change" clarifies what is going on here: When we attempt to change how we are and become different, that is, to be our true rather than conditioned self, we experience the fear of being rejected or abandoned by significant people and even by core-held subconscious beliefs for how we define ourselves, so much so that we stop from completing actions that will help us change to complete ourselves in desired ways. We develop an "immunity to change," a process that

keeps us the same rather than being able to change ourselves to be the way we want to be; we stay safe and do not
"trust" our ourselves to grow and become different and
more effective and complete as a unique person.

Kegan hypothesizes that we can develop a false sense of
self that for me prevents our working toward our sense of
completeness. He gives examples of when we act against
achieving a goal of improving ourselves, because changing
would mean giving up aspects of ourselves that are familiar
and safe, e.g., losing weight versus remaining comfortable
as we are; stopping procrastination versus facing head on
difficult challenges; changing an ineffective style of leadership versus relinquishing control over others; being more
open and sharing in our communication with others versus
remaining guarded and safe, etc. For Kegan, "giving ourselves a new form" involves changing or transforming our
meaning-making or the way we actively construct and re-
construct with our mind the understanding of reality and
our "authoring of the self."

In differentiating and integrating a new self we must
sometimes go against the self we have authored that is not
yet our true self. In "Immunity to Change," Kegan reinforces
the importance of supporting our meaning-making in service of growth and change. He offers us a process to use to
become more aware of how our "hidden competing com-
mitments" and related "big assumptions," resulting from
our history of learning how to be in the world, create an
"immunity to change" that prevents our reaching goals of
personal growth because we are not aware of learned habitual emotions that subconsciously keep us away from challenging ourselves. These learned ways of not being our true
self are deeply embedded feelings in our body that are

associated with our need to feel safe, e.g., eating makes me happy so in changing my eating habits to lose weight I must learn to change my emotional habit of eating to feel secure and happy.

This change is difficult, because we have to learn a different way of being, including thinking, behavior, and feelings, which often connect to fear of change. Kegan offers us "a more expansive way of knowing" to help us be more conscious or aware of how we stop ourselves from growing by avoiding emotions that we have learned to fear experiencing. In a related vein, Carl Rogers, one of the founders of Humanistic Psychology, notes in "Freedom to Learn" that "Learning, which involves a change in self-organization in the perception of oneself — is threatening and tends to be resisted." I see this resistance as the immunity to change. So, if we are to achieve completeness as a person, we must become knowledgeable about and squarely face our immunity to change!

I offer an example of a twenty-year-old Latina who in trying to determine what direction to take in college, including what college to attend. She is coming face-to-face with her immunity to change. She wants to make her own choices, but she is confronted by the wishes of what her family thinks is best for her and even a deeper commitment to be the way, maintain the self, who she has always been, in this case a person who has not developed her independent, autonomous self within her family.

This young woman recounted to me that in her childhood and adolescence she was constantly compared to her other family members and told she wasn't good enough and that she should be more like others. Now at twenty, she is struggling to become free from comparing herself and continuing to make herself the way her family wants her to be versus becoming who she wants to be. She speaks of the need to achieve her "deeper self," which I see is akin to defining her center, her core, her true self. She's searching to define who she really is. Her "immunity to change," the emotions of need for security and love that go with being part of her family, and the fear, doubt, and shame associated with going against her family, as well as her fear of experiencing change, are emotions which stop her from supporting her need to be true to herself, her immunity to change.

Also, she is coming directly in contact with her fear of doing something new and different because it may not work, she "may not work," just like she has been reminded over and over by her family. To continue the process of completing herself, she must face and master the fearful emotions associated with taking actions to support herself to be who she wants to be, to recognize both the importance of her family's love and support as well as her own self-love, that is, respect and support for her need to be an independent person. She must change her "self-organization!"

The fear of growth that Kegan addresses in the "Immunity to Change" is a theme related to personality development that I first came across in Abraham Maslow's book "Toward a Psychology of Being." This is a wonderful book where Maslow developed the optimistic ideas of Humanistic Psychology in contrast to what he considered the less optimistic ideas of human growth put forth by the psychoanalytic theory of Sigmund Freud and B. F. Skinner's behavior theory. Freud's theory posited that we have an animal nature that is always at war with societal norms and rules. Freud claimed that this process is primarily out of our awareness, that is, unconscious. Our hope as humans,

according to Freud, is to constantly work to become aware
of and to do our best to curb animal drives such as sex and
aggression. This struggle between our instinctual selves
(what Freud called "id") and conscious self (Freud's "ego"),
is a life challenge, according to Freud, where our only hope
is to constantly work to not give in to our unconscious desires, e.g., for sex and power. In contrast, Skinner argued
that all that we are and can become is determined by events
in our environment, rewards and punishments. These shape
who we are. Our mind and our ability to think are not as
important as rewards and punishments in our environment
that determine our actions and make us who we are.

Against Freud and Skinner's theories, Maslow developed
the notion that we are free to choose and direct our futures
and that we are naturally predisposed to grow and develop
our best possible self, which he called "self-actualization."
What was valuable for me in Maslow's work is his idea that
we can be guided by three different types of motivation: Deficiency motivation, maintenance motivation, and actualization motivation. Underlying these forms of motivation is
"The Need to Know versus The Fear of Knowing." While
we all have a natural or intrinsic drive to actualize our best
self, to know and be our real self, we also experience anxiety
when we try to do something different to what we've grown
accustomed to, especially when our actions threaten to separate us from the love and support of the world around us.

Deficiency motivation is when we act to be safe, to avoid
the possible disapproval of others or the threats of our social
and physical world. Maintenance motivation is when we
"stay in our own lane"- we stay safe and at the same we
avoid being different. Actualization motivation is when we
trust ourselves to act according to what we think is best both

for us and the world around us. We are interdependent; we don't enslave ourselves to others nor solely to our own ego needs. I have concluded from Maslow's work that to be complete as a human being is to grow beyond our fears, doubts, etc., to understand and manage our anxieties, and to choose to direct our development as a person towards being true to how we see the world.

À la Kegan and Maslow, the challenge of freeing ourselves to move toward becoming complete as persons has been clearly brought home to me by Ken Keyes' work "The Handbook to Higher Consciousness." I have read, reread, and taken long walks with this book for many, many hours, moment-by-moment developing a greater understanding about what it means for me to be a complete person. Keyes' ideas center around twelve pathways that we can take to develop ourselves. These pathways are related to increasingly attaining more developed centers of higher consciousness.

The first three pathways are grouped together under the rubric "Freeing Myself." Freeing self from what? (1) Security, sensation, and power addictions that keep me from loving myself and others; (2) Not being aware of how my consciousness-dominating addictions create my illusory version of the changing world around me; (3) Addictions I must re-program to free myself from my robot-like emotional patterns. Being conscious and acting on these three pathways, which Keyes recommends that we commit to memory, begin to liberate us, as Keyes writes, from our "dead past and our imagined future."

Memorizing the pathways is important for Keyes because doing so keeps these ideas in the forefront of our thinking, feeling, and behaving. I agree wholeheartedly! I have personally experienced the power of committing these principles to memory so as to psychologically be more complete, because the ideas become guides that we can hold in our minds and that we think about when faced with a challenging decision and related emotional trials to change our behavior.

The nine Keyes' pathways that follow are organized into three groups: Being Here and Now; Interacting with Others; and, finally, Discovering My Conscious-awareness. The first group emphasizes the power of being present in the here-and-now so that we can continuously work on our development. The next group defines how to be open and honest with others so as to constantly support our realities and truth as individuals. The final group emphasizes paying attention to freeing ourselves of our conditioned way of being to become aware of the peace and beauty that goes with simply focusing on awareness of the world and universe of which we are part. The last group includes Pathway 10: "I am continually calming the restless scanning of my rational mind in order to perceive the finer energies that enable me to intuitively merge with everything around me."

In reading and rereading "The Pathway to Higher Consciousness," I have again come to the notion that to become complete is to develop, grow, change, from a person who is governed by outside forces to a person who trusts and supports his or her mind to guide self to "*Saber, Entender, Sentir, Escoger y Hacer*," the person that one truly wants to be — to complete one's understanding of all the possibilities and growth that life offers!

The notion of "trusting and supporting self" is a factor related to completing self that I have seen come up over and over again in psychological literature, but no more forcefully than in the writing and thinking of Erik Erikson.

Erikson wrote a famous book titled "Childhood and Society," wherein he separated from Freud's notion of unconscious forces that dominate our existence to the idea that as humans we develop unique strengths and virtues through our social-psychological interactions with others. For Erikson, the "virtues" we develop as we live life are "strengths" that support our psychological growth. This happens as we go through eight stages of development: Trust versus Mistrust (first year); Autonomy versus Shame and Doubt (two to three years); Initiative versus Guilt (ages four to five); Industry versus inferiority (beginning school years); Identity versus Role Confusion (adolescence); Intimacy versus Isolation (beginning in adulthood); Generativity versus Stagnation (our adult career years); Ego Integrity versus Despair (coming to the end of our life).

The virtues/strengths that individuals develop during these periods, which Erikson clarifies after his initial book "Childhood and Society," are the following: Hope; will power; purpose; competence; fidelity; love; care, wisdom. Erikson's stages are each characterized by social psychological challenges to a person's development. Resolution of these challenges with support from others and progressively with more and more support from self leads to greater ego development of the person, which is the ability to define and direct one's personal identity and understanding of self in the world.

The beauty of Erikson's book, a challenging book which was the first significant book on psychology that I read not as an academic assignment, is that it is a useful summary of Erikson's ideas on what it means to develop one's identity as a human being. With respect to offering me and the world what it means to be complete as a person, I see Erikson's work as providing another roadmap for challenges individuals face to realize themselves as unique persons. We are social beings, and, as such, we must understand how our social-psychological selves are subject to forces that can turn us away from trusting ourselves to think and be who we are versus giving up this most human of characteristics. For example, we can develop trust versus mistrust, autonomy versus shame and doubt, etc., and each challenge either brings us closer to being and completing our self or results in separation from the self.

Related to clarifying the ideas of Erik Erikson, I recommend a short book by Dr. Richard Evans of the University of Houston, wherein Evans has a dialogue with Erikson regarding Erikson's ideas related to the eight stages of social-psychological development. I love this book because Erikson responds to questions from Dr. Evans in a simple and clear manner. The way Erikson talks about the power of developing the virtue of hope out of the challenge of trust versus mistrust is one example. Erikson speaks: "Hope is a very basic human strength without which we couldn't stay alive," to which Erikson cites the work of Spitz who studied thousands of children in orphanages who did not get enough contact from caretakers, where "children give up hope because they do not get enough loving and stimulation (and) may literally die." The children became listless and non-responsive to others, thereby lessening their chances to learn from others and to receive the love of others.

And, Erikson adds that hope is not built up solely in the first year of life as a result of the relation between mother and infant, "but that because of lifelong struggles between trust and mistrust in changing states and conditions, it [hope] has to be developed firmly, and then be confirmed and reaffirmed throughout life." (Evans, 1967). This book is significant with respect to what it means to be complete as a person because Erikson provides another roadmap for what it means to develop one's uniqueness as a person. My takeaway from Erikson is that to be complete we again change, grow, and develop throughout life, and, importantly, that our process of change and growth depends on how much trust versus mistrust we have toward others, but most especially toward ourselves.

I have always looked to books that detail the insights of sages and what they can teach me, especially related to completing myself as a person. One such book is Rick Hanson and Richard Mendius' "Buddha's Brain: The Practical Neuroscience of Happiness, Love and Wisdom." I was first introduced to the authors in a workshop given by them at the Spirit Rock Meditation Center in Woodacre, California. I went there with a wonderful Latina friend, and the day was peaceful and informative. Hanson and Mendius' book, however, went far beyond the workshop, providing me with a broad introduction to cognitive neuroscience, especially how what the authors termed the "self-transforming brain," coupled with knowledge of how Buddhist meditative practices can help us live more peaceful, loving and effective lives.

The book moves from a review of the how the evolutionary biological nature of our central nervous system (brain and spinal cord) and our endocrine system (our glands and hormones), and how as a result of our human evolution we have a dual nature that is on the "edge of a sword" between fear and anxiety and "happiness, peace and love." With a review of basic cognitive-neuroscience information at the front of the book, the authors share how our brains have evolved the ability to flexibly adapt to the changing demands of our environment.

The latter is known as neuroplasticity wherein the billions of our neurons, communication cells in the brain and spinal cord, have given us the ability to change our way of living so as to better adapt to life. The authors apply this knowledge to "Taking in the Good," "Strong Intentions," and "Equanimity," chapters that teach us how to internalize the positives in our lives, strengthen our motivation, and cool the fires of greed, hatred, and delusion by learning to steady our mind through increased mindfulness and meditative practice.

Hanson and Medius' work has helped me further understand what it means for me to become complete as a human being: I need to understand how I am a biological-psychological person; I must know how my mind and body as a unified organism works and how I can either "incline my mind toward the positive," or let my less evolved instincts of greed, hatred, and delusion control my life. One of the most powerful chapters in "Buddha's Brain" is the chapter entitled the "First and Second Dart." This chapter covers how an unchecked Sympathetic Nervous System (our fight or flight system) and our Hypothalamic-Pituitary-Adrenal Axis (SNS/HPAA), our system of glands and hormones that are responsible for supporting our ongoing response to stress by releasing cortisol and adrenaline, can lead to anxiety and depression, and, how, if we follow a "Path of Practice," we can become "awake persons" who can correct and direct our biological-psychological life toward the positive and away from the negative.

The "Path of Practice" is a four-step process whereby we first become aware of how we habitually and negatively respond to challenges for growth in life to developing a progressively more positive response to life's stresses where we learn to be calm, and eventually to progress through life's challenges without burdening our biopsychological system with damaging stress responses. In "Buddha's Brain," I found that evolution has provided humans with an integrated organism that has an organization of nearly 100 billion neurons that all support us to live in a complete and joyful manner. We only have to learn how to trust and use our biology to complete our personality with "happiness, love, and wisdom."

I have always been fascinated by what factors affect the development of personality. This clearly relates to persons becoming complete because our personal identity directs our efforts to become and complete who we are. It is important to ask how our personality can help or hinder our efforts to develop a cohesive, unified and complete self. Eric Berne's book, "Transactional Analysis," provides some answers to this question. Berne recounts experiments where a person's feeling and thinking states from past memories can be elicited directly by stimulation of the brain. Yes, a person can literally repeat earlier memories in the manner that they initially experienced simply through the electrical stimulation of certain parts of the brain! The brain is like a computer that stores information, and the information when appropriately "stimulated" by life events can be reexperienced in response to ongoing situations in the environment.

Berne theorized three "ego states" related to past memories recorded in our brain. These "ego states" characterize personality factors that influence adult thinking, feeling, and behaving. Berne gave these ego-states specific names: Parent, Adult, and Child. This idea helped me think about how we can support or not support ourselves to become complete. According to Berne, ego states "form a coherent system of feelings related to a given subject and preferred ways of behaving (a set of behavior patterns, e.g., attention, liking, excited body, etc.) that direct persons to act based more on emotional patterns of behavior rather than actions based on information-based logical reasoning." The ego states of Parent and Child are preserved (cathected) in memory in childhood and are activated as "scripts" in adult behavior. Scripts are preordained ways of responding to life situations. The outcome is that very often Parent and Child pre-ordained "tapes" guide behavior automatically and are not based on reasoned judgement.

The usefulness of Berne's theory of personality is that we are able to become aware of the dynamics of our personality organization and so can learn to choose to change ineffective "scripts" through a form of therapy or learning called "Transactional Analysis (TA)." When reading Berne's book, I became more aware of how I learned to think, feel, and behave in very automatic ways in childhood. I became more aware of how my adult thinking, feelings, and behavior were like recorded transcripts from my past. I could see myself as an adult acting out certain mannerisms (e.g., tone of voice, body gestures, and facial expressions) that I had learned very early in childhood, and I became more aware of how my "Child" thinking and behavior habits prevented me from developing into the person I wanted to be.

I have learned that effective functioning involves understanding Parent and Child scripts and learning to use the Adult ego state to change ineffective and habitual scripts. The Child ego state is that aspect of the self that demands gratification and is self-focused, whereas the Parent ego state directs the individual to do what is right and correct according to moral, cultural or societal principles literally passed down from parents and society. The Child ego state is learned early in childhood based on experiences with key others, e.g., parents, family members, etc. The Parent ego state, in turn, is learned primarily in interaction with the parents, wherein the parents' beliefs and rules are taken on as "shoulds."

These "should-isms," in turn, direct the individual's actions in a preordained or mechanical manner, e.g., "I should do this; I should think a certain way," etc. Problems in personality development in adulthood occur when the Parent and Child ego states overwhelm the personality. Transactional Analysis supports the individual to free the self from sub-conscious scripts of the Parent and Child and to use the Adult ego state, that aspect of the psychological self that can use rational logic to make effective choices that integrate all aspects of the individual's psychology as well as reality-based information from the physical and social world in such a way as to direct us to make life choices and take actions in a reasoned and constructive manner.

I use the ideas of TA to educate people how the structure of personality can be influenced by how we've characteristically developed scripts that make use of the Parent and Child roles. I share that ego states are memories in our brains that literally can turn on automatically in their almost original form in response to life challenges. As is the goal in TA, learning about one's personality structure can help us be more aware of how our past learning influences present behavior, and we can become more capable to direct the development of our personality in a logical and reasoned manner.

The idea of becoming who you really are is an idea of TA that I especially share with others. In this regard, in TA there is a contrast in personality functioning between the "real or authentic self" and "not real self." The "real self" functions effectively in the world using evidence to understand the "data" of reality and limits the use of Child and Parent "shoulds," and chooses effective ways of behaving that support the unique psychological growth of the individual. A major aspect of TA is to learn to monitor how in interaction with others our and their use or non-use of Parent, Child, and Adult ego states help or hinder our growth as individuals.

There is another book, "I'm OK — You're OK" by Thomas Harris, M.D., that is a more readable version of the concepts and use of Transactional Analysis for improved personality development. I have found this book to be more practical for laypersons to understand and use TA principles. One of the most useful aspects of Dr. Harris' book is that he frames the concepts of Parent, Adult, and Child as being expressed in one of "four life positions" that are learned early in life: I'm not OK — You're OK; I'm OK — You're not OK; I'm not OK — You're not OK; I'm OK — You're OK.

Harris hypothesizes that in the first two years of life we generally learn the I'm not OK — You're OK position, because we can do so little on our own, and as one-to-two-year-old children, we are frustrated by the many limits we have in accessing our environments as well as from difficulties we have when experiencing different types of parenting styles, especially what I would call unsupportive parents, e.g., unloving parents, overly disciplining parents, etc. When parents are unsupportive of us, we learn the "I'm not

OK" position. According to Harris, the four life positions are initially developed in the first five years of life, but can be changed through life experience.

Harris covers how the TA concepts relate to the four life positions. For me, here lies the power of Harris' book. He clearly describes how the learning of scripts can affect how we think about the psychological dynamics within ourselves as well as between ourselves and others, and he outlines how we can develop our psychological selves by learning "How to Stay in the Adult." Again, the power of TA for me is that we can use its principles to understand ourselves and how we support or limit our growth as persons. Harris' words are useful here:

"The Adult develops later than the Parent and Child and seems to have a difficult time catching up throughout life. The Parent and Child occupy primary circuits (memories in brain), which tend to come on automatically in response to stimuli. The first way, therefore, to build the strength of the Adult is to become sensitive to Parent and Child signals. Aroused feelings are a clue that the Child has been hooked. To know one's own Child, to be sensitive to one's own Not OK feelings, is the first requirement for Adult data (information) processing. Being aware of, "That is my NOT OK Child," makes it possible to keep externalizing the feelings in actions. Processing this data takes a moment. Counting to ten is a useful way to delay the automatic response in order that the Adult maintain control of the transaction. "When in doubt, leave it out" is a good practice." (Page 92).

Harris provides practical "clues" to recognizing when we are moving into the Child or Parent ego states — to know one's Child or Parent self. Also, Harris provides guides for how to limit the strength of the Parent and Child ego states in our life. For example, one of the insights I gained was that an important strength of the Adult ego state is the ability to show restraint: "In restraining the automatic, archaic responses of Parent and Child, while waiting for the Adult to compute appropriate responses." Another insight for developing the Adult ego state in our personality is that "conscious effort is required to make big decisions," and to do this it is important to work out a value system to guide our decision-making. When we have a thoroughly developed value system, we are less prone to the automatic, emotional thinking and acting of the Parent and Child selves.

Harris offers the following as a summary of how to build a strong Adult self:

- Learn to recognize your Child, its vulnerabilities, its fears, its principal methods of expressing these feelings;
- Learn to recognize your Parent, its admonitions, injunctions, fixed positions, and principal ways of expressing these admonitions, injunctions, positions;
- Count to ten, if necessary, in order to give the Adult time to process the data coming into the computer (our brain), to sort out Parent and Child from reality;
- When in doubt, leave it out. You can't be attacked for what you didn't say;
- Work out a system of values. You can't make decisions without an ethical framework.

So, using the ideas of Transactional Analysis, we can conclude that to complete ourselves, we must become conscious of the automatic or sub-conscious forces that direct our behaviors.

Before leaving this section, I want to share some ideas

related to our becoming complete from a book called "Body-wise" by Joseph Heller and William A. Henkin. I had the pleasure in 2015 to spend a week doing "bodywork" with Joseph Heller at his office at the foot of Mt. Shasta, California. Heller took me through a series of body learning steps wherein I became more aware of how my body reflected my psychology, what I have seen referred to as biopsychology. The essence of the work is detailed in the book "Bodywise," wherein we are taught about how in life we learn to hold our body in ineffective ways, and, in short, these attitudes of the body become what I would call our unbalanced personality. How do we change this lack of balance? We change by learning that our body (bones, muscles, tendons, etc.,) has a natural unified balance that is meant to accompany us through our life experiences, but that this balance can become disturbed by negative psychological experiences:

"Whenever we feel unstable we tense up (or compress) somewhere in our bodies. By doing this we achieve exactly the opposite of what we intended: Instead of making ourselves more stable we make ourselves less stable. The feeling of instability that makes us tense up need not be physical. Although walking a shaky plank over a high chasm will bring the lesson home immediately and impressively, it can be derived equally well from feelings of psychological or mental instability, as Wilhelm Reich, Lowen, and others have pointed out. Gripping psychologically or mentally can lead to emotional and mental rigidities in the same way that gripping physically leads to physical rigidities. *Moreover, physical rigidities lead to psychological rigidities, and psychological rigidities lead to physical rigidities (mine).* Because the human being is an integrated system, gripping in any realm will affect stability in *every* realm. This is easiest to see, of course, and easiest to address, in the body." (Page 130).

"Bodywise" is a book which teaches us about the way our bodies naturally should be aligned and balanced to support our daily lives. We also learn and see how our bodies and minds, our biological-psychological selves, can be misaligned. We also learn in this special book how different "body traditions" have evolved to help us understand, align, and balance our biopsychological selves. Ideas and methods to balance and integrate our biopsychological selves are shared from authors such as Wilhelm Reich, Stanley Keleman, Alexander Lowen, Ida Rolf, and Moshe Feldenkrais, wherein we learn that there are different perspectives for how to reestablish the integrity and effective functioning of a united body and mind.

A major part of "Bodywise" is to introduce us to the specific methods of Hellerwork, wherein a person is taken through ten sessions to learn his or her body as well as to learn to begin reestablishing the balance and oneness of our biopsychological selves. The following is a general description of the Hellerwork and reason behind the bodywork of each session:

- Inspiration (releasing our upper body so as to take in the necessary oxygen for a healthy life);
- Understanding or standing on your own two feet (learning how our feet are naturally meant to have balance to support our whole body as well as how to reinitiate this balance);
- Reaching out (how we can be effective "leaning into life," using our arms and bodies in effective ways so as to express personal initiative and direction);

- Surrender and control (learning how to release tension and gripping so as to develop more trust in ourselves);
- Gut feelings, holding back, and losing your head (learning to trust our natural instincts in reaching out and interacting with others);
- Feminine and masculine energy (learning to be receptive toward our feminine and masculine selves);
- Integration and coming out (clarifying and beginning to practice new attitudes and manners to express our biopsychological selves in an integrated and unified manner).

Gestalt Books Related to Becoming a Complete Person

My goal, to repeat, pure and simple, is to get you to read, learn from, and use Gestalt books and other psychological literature to support your efforts to complete yourself as close as possible to what you want. So, let's look at Gestalt books that have fascinated me and that have led me to pick them up over and over again to gain a deeper understanding of the themes of my personality and support me becoming my "real self." I see the "real self" as equivalent to the "complete self." Still, questions remain as to what these ideas mean, especially from a Gestalt perspective. Let's start from the grand promoter of Gestalt therapy, Fritz Perls. In "Gestalt Therapy Verbatim," what I consider to be a fascinating book, Perls shares how he sees the idea of completeness:

> "No one of us is complete . . . every one of us has holes in his personality . . . Where something should be, there is nothing. Many people have no soul. Others have no genitals. Some have no heart; all their

energy goes into computing, thinking. Others have no
legs to stand on. Many people have no eyes. They
project the eyes, and the eyes are to quite an extent in
the outside world and always live as if they are being
looked at [similar to what I have heard from many
Latin@ students *"pienso que todos me estan mirando"*].
A person feels that the eyes of the world are upon
him. He becomes a mirror-person who always wants
to use his eyes to see how he looks to others. He gives
up his eyes and asks the world to do his seeing for
him. Instead of being critical, he projects the criticism
and feels criticized and feels on stage . . . Now the
most important missing part is the center . . . This
achieving the center, being grounded in one's self, is
about the highest state a human being can achieve.

"No one is complete?" This speaks clearly to me about
myself as well as for many of the thousands of persons I
have taught and counseled. What comes to mind are all
those situations when I have not stood up for myself: When
others were negating my experience of my "true self," when
I have not spoken up because I was afraid of being rejected
for being different, and when I did not act on a desire because I was embarrassed to own my true self. When I was
embarrassed to be seen!

We all seek completeness, but we all have "unfinished
business," "incomplete Gestalts and holes" in our personality. Perls wrote that, "The average person of our time, believe it or not, lives only 5 percent of his potential available."
Really, only 5 percent? I'll leave the possible reality of this
statement to each of us to determine how much we live up
to our potential, and, as such, I am being true to the Gestalt
idea that it is we as individuals who define and create our

experience of becoming complete as persons. In this regard, Fritz Perls noted that Gestalt therapy (and what I have expanded to call personal development work) is phenomenological, which mean that the work done is based on an individual's "firsthand experiencing" of self. Basically, defining our level of completeness comes down to being aware of how we act, and, importantly, being aware of how we perceive and experience ourselves.

So, what about the holes Perls talks about? Simply stated, they are incomplete Gestalts, as Perls writes: "Our life is nothing but a series of incomplete Gestalts." To me, incomplete Gestalts connect to experiences where we do not complete the Gestalt Cycle of Experience, which Joseph Zinker so artfully describes in his book "The Creative Process in Gestalt Therapy."

"As work progresses, the person flows more comfortably in the experience of his energy and uses it in a way which allows him completeness of functioning. He acts without dissipating his energy by learning to creatively integrate conflicting feelings within himself, rather than pushing against his own organism."

And how do we fill in the holes in our personality and complete "incomplete Gestalts/unfinished business?" This is done by adhering to the "awareness principle," which means practicing our natural ability to be conscious/aware of our inner and outer experiences. Perls wrote that, "awareness by itself is curative." In fact, awareness is a central tenet of what Perls called "Organismic Self-Regulation." To have health is to "have a balance and coordination of what we are — a human organism". We are billions of cells all working in the service of our living and adapting to life. If we learn to trust our organism, we will be able to move toward the completeness of that which we are. Perls wrote:

"So, we come to our basic conflict and the basic conflict is this: Every individual, every plant, every animal has only one inborn goal — to actualize itself as it is. A rose is a rose is a rose. A rose is not intent to actualize itself as a kangaroo. An elephant is not intent to actualize itself as a bird. In nature — except for human beings, constitution and healthiness, potential, growth, is all one unified something."

Let's spend a little time looking at one of the main reasons why we are unable to become a unified whole, what Perls alludes to as having holes in our personality. We have seen that coordinating and expressing a unified personality is an important Gestalt principle. But this is generally not the case, as most of us tend think and act in a non-integrated and non-unified way; we may think and feel in one way, and act in a way inconsistent with our thinking and feeling. Why? Because our development as individuals is too often fraught with experiences where we think, feel, and act against ourselves because our environment, family, friends, school authorities, etc., demand this of us and generally do not support development of our unique self.

We too often are not sufficiently powerful to stand up for ourselves, hold our space, especially during the vulnerable time of childhood, so we develop incomplete Gestalts, holes and unfinished business, where rather than self-expression we learn shame, embarrassment, fear, avoidance, and often, self-rejection. These make up the holes in our personality. Our ability to perceive, think, and act as we deem correct is replaced by what Robert G. Lee calls "shame binds." Wheeler defines this process in his chapter "Shame and the

Gestalt Model," in the book "The Voice of Shame" edited by Lee and Gordon Wheeler:

"The experience of shame occurs whenever in life, especially during the vulnerable time of childhood, when we reach out in hope to meet our needs but, instead, we experience shame, which is the experience that what is me is not acceptable, that this is not my world. As such, shame signifies a rupture (or a threat of rupture) between the individual's needs and goals on the one hand and environmental receptivity to those needs and goals on the other ... and ... the need that is not received by the other is disowned and made 'not me'."

So, we come to a clearer understanding that the holes in our personality and our unfinished business require mending. The holes or splits in our personality, what we experience as "me-not me," have been created by experiences where we have not resolved our need to use "self-support" to meet our needs and satisfy our wants. Instead, we have avoided our natural function to act and complete situations to meet what we deem desirable. Gestalt work is a process of filling in the holes, splits in our personality, again, by focusing and paying attention and working on completing the unfinished business in our present moment, e.g., use of the empty chair technique which I introduced in Chapter 2 which allows us to revitalize and reintegrate a more complete self.

Irving and Miriam Polster, in their excellent book "Gestalt Therapy Integrated," allude to the process of filling in the holes in our personality or completing our unfinished business:

"Whenever unfinished business forms the center of one's existence, one's effervescence of mind becomes hampered. Ideally, the unencumbered person is free to engage spontaneously with whatever interests him and to stay with it until this lively interest subsides and something else draws his attention. This is a natural process and a person who lives according to this rhythm experiences himself as flexible, clear, and effective."

Aha! Unfinished business can form the center of our existence! Here is where Perls emphasizes the idea that all of us have a center to direct our actions. With this center we can be grounded in the experience of our self and we can have "balance" and we can "facilitate the development of authentic growth." We can, as noted by the Polsters, "live . . . flexible, clear, and effective lives!"

So, I arrive at a formal statement for the meaning of "It is our birthright to achieve completeness." Evolution has brought us to the point of being able to be aware of our own process of being, and "our senses and accompanying perceptions are the means of awareness, consciousness, attention." Being complete means that we are a unified, integrated, sentient organism (responsive to or conscious of sense impressions) where the center of our organism is the "self-in-action." This self can be framed as a process of organizing and authoring a self; and, this self can be framed as a developmental process of growth that moves through different stages of awareness, e.g., emotional, cognitive, behavioral, biopsychological, universal spirituality.

https://youtu.be/3_OoFoGSvBw
**Link to me doing Gestalt work with Joseph Zinker,
clarifying my journey to completeness**

Again, the self we are and seek to complete can be diverted or subverted depending on how our environment supports or does not support our development of clarity in defining and being our real, authentic, and true self. This is a truth relevant to each of our searches for completeness. Will Schutz, in his powerful book "The Human Element," identifies "truth as the great equalizer" as the main factor that supports us knowing and being effective with ourselves and others. As such, I see supporting our efforts toward being complete means constantly clarifying what is truth for each of us. Importantly, clarifying truth means being in contact with the positive flow of energy in our bodies as we experience truth. As such, with our whole organism we react and respond to life to provide greater clarity or truth of who we are and what we want, and we use "self-expression" to realize or complete our self.

In summary, barring biological abnormalities, we are all born with an organism exquisitely evolved to be able to be aware of our needs and wants and to use our five senses, to use the 100 billion of our communication cells, our neurons, to interact with the environment to meet what we determine as necessary for an effective and satisfying life. In this process, we all have ongoing experiences that emerge, stand out (so-called emergencies in Gestalt), that communicate to us the need to be aware and act in accordance to what we experience as a whole and unified self — our truth. When we act from our center, from our "real self," we experience "contact" with who we are, and, at the same time, we define what is "not me." We live out our birthright to be complete, which is exquisitely defined in the Gestalt Cycle of Experience: Sensation, Awareness, Mobilization of Energy, Action, Contact, Assimilation, and Withdrawal.

Before leaving this section, I want to briefly mention other Gestalt books that have essential insights regarding what it means to be complete. Each of these books merit you reading them for greater understanding of how to meet the challenges of your personal development. For example, in Muriel Schiffman's heartfelt book "Gestalt Self Therapy," she writes the following in the chapter titled "Search for Identity:"

"To be an authentic person is to know who you really are, to experience the conflicting sides of your personality. Self-therapy (and especially Gestalt self-therapy) is a path to self-knowledge . . . When you reach a hidden facet of yourself and realize how you have been lying to yourself and others all these years, you may begin to feel ashamed. This is the time to remember that you did not invent this system of defenses out of thin air, just for fun. You developed this system in childhood in order to survive . . . A whole person is three-dimensional, a complex bundle of traits. The in-authentic person is artificial, two-dimensional, because in screening out one side of an inner conflict he exaggerates the other. He is a caricature of a whole person."

With a steady, firm, and loving hand, Schiffman guides us to steadfastly stick with our efforts to face the difficult challenges that are part of knowing and being our real self. She over and over challenges us to dig deep into the "splits" within our personality wherein occurs the battle between non-self-support and self-support. In doing this, Schiffman shares her own life journey and themes, all the while modeling the courage needed to face and change and develop ourselves for the better.

Another important Gestalt book, edited by John O. Stevens, is titled "Gestalt Is." Twelve authors share their insights to the power of Gestalt personal development concepts, but, as always, I am drawn to the writings of Fritz Perls in the chapter entitled "Theory and Technique of Personality Integration:"

'Integration, in the final analysis, is prevented by the desensitization of the emotional barriers, especially the disgust, embarrassment, shame, anxiety, and fear barriers . . . We have not only the task to expose them, but we also have to turn them into cooperative energies . . . Disgust turns via greed into discrimination (ability to see different perspectives); anxiety via excitement into specific interest, such as hostility, sexual excitement, enthusiasm, initiative, etc.; fear via suspicion into experimentation; and embarrassment via exhibitionism into self-expression . . . (all this in service of reaching) a state of integration (unity of self) which facilitates its own development."

Wow! There's so much to understand in Perls' words, but the short of it is that if we are to be able to assume more complete responsibility for our lives — our thinking, feeling, and behaving — we must get to know ourselves (*Saber, Entender*), and feel ourselves (*Sentir*), so as to be able to choose and act (*Escoger y Hacer*) who we really are.

Summarizing Chapter 9 and Moving Forward to Chapter 10, Where I will Introduce a Practical Method for Organizing the Search for Completeness

The following are key concepts from the books I have introduced related to the upcoming chapter. There I will present a method that I have developed, "The 0-100% Circle of Development," to help you to identify what factors you see as important to achieve completeness. An important idea related to becoming complete as a person is that all of us continually develop psychologically through our lifespan.

I have included Robert Kegan's notion that we experience ongoing change in the way we think and feel about our self, ranging from a position with no understanding or perception of the self (Incorporative Self and Impulsive Self), to a gradual evolution of our meaning-making self, where we organize a clear sense of who we are in relation to others, and finally, a self who sees the need to have a balanced interaction with others (The Interindividual Balance). The central process that Kegan communicates to us is a movement where first we are what he calls an "embeddual," with limited clarity of perception regarding our existence to progressively becoming an individual. As an "embeddual," we do not have a clear experience that we have senses and reflexes; rather, we are embedded in our senses and reflexes.

With progressively improved "meaning-making," we free ourselves from simply "being our senses and reflexes" to the point when we are able to experience that we have a self who uses our senses and reflexes to interact with the world. We begin to become an individual by accommodating or changing our experience of our self in the world. Again, we progressively learn to understand that we construct or make meaning of our unique experiences. What happens is that we begin to understand that our development as an individual is not automatic, but requires effort. We learn that sometimes we can lessen our growth by continuing with habitual ways of being because we are fearful of change. We become fearful of letting go of our past self, which is often based on our need to feel safe.

Kegan calls this our "immunity to change." If we challenge ourselves, we can learn to change what I might call a "safe attitude toward self," a built-in defense mechanism to stop ourselves from experiencing anything that is fearful, different, and challenging. To get past our immunity to change, we need to use our self-awareness to detect how we avoid developing our potential. We must choose to author a self that we truly want. Abraham Maslow characterized this human process as, "the need to know versus the fear of knowing." Yes, we want to know and change, but we are afraid of the challenges that go with being truthful about who we are and how we don't support ourselves to improve as persons.

Erik Erikson offered that we can more effectively author our self by developing different psychological strengths, what he calls virtues, e.g., the strength of autonomy. He also noted that we can also develop psychological weaknesses through our lifespan, e.g., the weakness of shame and doubt. The beauty of Erikson is that he shows us how we develop strengths in our personality by resolving ongoing socio-psychological challenges. The most important challenge for Erikson is the development of "trust" in self and with others. This leads to the virtue of hope, which makes us more open and resilient to life. Importantly, the challenge of trust versus mistrust and the possible strengthening of hope, according to Erikson, are reexperienced time and again in our life when we face the need to trust ourselves and others so as to adapt more effectively to what we think and feel is the truth of our life. Again, the strengths we can develop over the lifespan range from trust, autonomy, initiative, industry (skillful self), identity, intimacy, generativity (caring for others), our clarity and acceptance of who we are, and our integrity. The weaknesses we can develop range from mistrust, shame and doubt, inferiority, role confusion, isolation, stagnation, and despair. In the end, the virtues support us to progressively work to have integrity or unity regarding the experience of our self.

Ken Keyes provides a pathway for how we can change our behavior to continue to build what I consider a more complete self. This more complete self would be what Keyes calls the development of a higher consciousness. For example, in the third pathway to higher consciousness, Keyes recommends that we memorize and remain vigilant to the act of managing our emotions to support positive growth: "I welcome the opportunity, even if painful, that my minute-to-minute experience offers me to become aware of the addictions (security, sensation, and power addictions) that I must reprogram to free myself of my robot-like emotional patterns." Freeing ourselves from our past is part of becoming complete, which eventually helps us to attain a higher level of completeness or higher consciousness. This freeing ourselves from our past is a theme that runs through all the books I have shared.

Carl Jung adds to the picture of what is our completeness by including the need to integrate our unconscious with our conscious self. Jung wrote that the psyche or self "exists to create more consciousness." This is accomplished by a person becoming more and more aware of how his/her personality is made up of both the conscious mind and the sub-conscious and unconscious aspects of the mind. The sub-conscious mind, which with effort is accessible to our awareness, is composed of information from an individual's life experiences that are hidden from the self, repressed, because they are too difficult to accept. Nevertheless, with Gestalt personal development work and other forms of therapy, we can progressively become more aware of our real self.

The Gestalt Cycle of Experience is a way of approaching experience to add more and more awareness for how we either support or not support our development of completeness as a unique person. In short, increased awareness of self, our motivations, fears, and desires, allows our natural inclination to actualize ourselves to occur. Awareness itself is curative, because our organism is geared to use awareness to choose how we truly want to be.

Dr. Rivas' Notes for Chapter 9:
Reviewing, repeating, realizing.

Although repetitive, I offer the following summaries of select author I have introduced to help you further understand the information:

- Kegan — "Person" refers to an activity of constantly giving ourselves a new form; we are meaning-makers, organizing, authoring our "self;" we progress through developmental stages in life that move from being "embedduals," where we are embedded in our limited perceptions of life developed as children, to become increasingly an individual who is aware of how we are separate from and are part of the social and physical world.

- Branden — Six foundational pillars of self-esteem, with "Living Consciously" being at the center. We can use six-pillar work to support our development of self-esteem.

- Maslow — The Need to Know versus the Fear of Knowing. We can have different motivations in life with respect to developing self-esteem: deficiency motivation; maintenance motivation; actualization motivation.

- Keyes — Important to memorize the definition of steps in the pathway to higher consciousness because it helps to keep focus. Pathway progresses from Freeing Self, to Being Here and Now, to Interacting with Others, and, finally, to Discovering My Conscious Awareness. This movement is from animal instincts to lower forms of ego-based consciousness to higher consciousness.

- Erikson — Eight Stages of Development wherein we develop strengths or virtues that support us to develop our social-psychological selves. The virtue of "Trust" is the primary strength that supports the healthy development of the self.

- Hanson and Mendius — Our biological inheritance bequeathed that we live on the edge of a sword between basic animal instincts and a conscious self who can exist as a unified organism with happiness, love, and wisdom.

- Bernes — We need to become knowledgeable of our "Child" and "Parent" ego states wherein we have "life scripts" that we develop in childhood. With this awareness we can develop our "real self." We can use Transactional Analysis (TA) to develop the reasoning, logical aspects of our "Adult" ego.

- Harris — There are four life positions that are related to

TA life scripts. These positions are: (1) I'm not OK; You're OK;" (2) "I'm Not OK; You're Not OK;" (3) I'm OK; You're Not OK;" (4) I'm OK; You're OK." Like Berne, Harris emphasizes that we can learn to disentangle ourselves from negative learning to develop our true self.

- Heller — "Bodywork" can help us integrate our physical and psychological selves. We lose the unity of who we are when our negative psychology rigidifies our physical self, and we lose flexibility.

- Perls — Develop the "real self" and facilitate authentic growth through the "awareness principle." Clear up holes in our personality, achieve a center, have balance.

- Polsters — Gestalt work supports the development of the "unencumbered person" who is free to engage spontaneously with life.

- Lee and Wheeler — We develop "shame binds" and a "voice of shame" when in early life we reach out for acceptance and support and experience rejection. We can withdraw or pull back from reaching out and "leaning into" life.

- Schiffman — We can do self-therapy to become aware and change the "hidden facets" of ourselves, and thereby heal the "splits" in our personality.

Chapter 10

Professional Development: The 0-100% Competence Model and Circle of Development- A Practical Approach to Organize and Monitor Progress For Becoming Complete as a Person

As is readily apparent from the unlimited number of published books about personal development, becoming complete as a person is a broad and challenging topic. In this chapter I will share how I help individuals approach understanding and becoming complete in a practical and organized way. By practical, I mean a way that one can organize the different developmental challenges of everyday life: What skills do I need to be successful in my career? What personality characteristics are required of me to interact effectively with others, etc. In this chapter, I also connect how I conceptualize a connection between the 0-100% Competence Model and Gestalt personal development in what I call "The Zone of Growth or Change." Finally, I also share how I have searched out my own completeness as a professional, especially someone whose value is to support other's personal growth.

In 1988, after a challenging nine years of on-and-off study, I completed my Doctor of Philosophy degree in Counseling and Student Personnel Psychology at the University of Minnesota, Minneapolis (U of M). In my dissertation, I formally introduced the concept of the "0-100% Competence Model," a way of structuring and monitoring skill development. During my doctoral studies, I worked full-time at the Martin Luther King Advising Program in the College of Liberal Arts (CLA) at the U of M. At the end of my tenure at the MLK Program, I was Assistant Director, and my most important work was to assist advisors and tutors to support the success of MLK students, most of whom were African American and Latin@. I developed the "0-100% Competence Model" to help students be organized and specific about improving their academic and personal development skills. In retrospect, this model was an expression of my ideas about how a person moves toward becoming complete as a unique individual.

Students liked the "0-100 % Competence Model" because it was simple to understand and straightforward to apply. It gave them a clear look at where they perceived their standing on a specific skill or personality characteristic that they needed for success in university studies, e.g., skills such as college-level writing, mathematics, and reading; characteristics such as self-discipline, time management, being organized, taking care of one's physical health; personality traits such as assertiveness, conscientiousness, agreeableness, etc. Essentially, students could use the 0-100% scale to identify the level of skill they perceived necessary to possess in school, career, or personal development characteristics, and could choose a numerical achievement goal on the scale, e.g., "To be competent in college I need to develop my reading skill to a level of 80 out of 100." One important aspect of students' development to which I applied the 0-100% scale was related to understanding how an individual's perceived skill ratings affected achievement motivation.

From a perspective of developing my work as a professional counselor and educator, use of the 0-100% scale, however, was not my first effort at finding a method to challenge and support students to be clear about their actual skill level as well as need for improvement. Arriving at the 0-100% scale was part of the process of study and application of research. I had come upon the idea of using a numerical scale to help students be more effective in planning their skill and personal development efforts as a result of my study in the area of achievement motivation, specifically the theorizing of Dr. John Atkinson of Purdue University. Atkinson pioneered the use of mathematical formulas to understand motivation and achievement. For example, he used a 0 to 1.0 scale to define a person's motivation, e.g., .3, .4, etc. Atkinson theorized that motivation toward a task was inverse to the level of difficulty of a task, e.g., if a task was .9 difficult, motivation would be low .1.

I can imagine that as you read this you may think as I did when I first read Atkinson's ideas, "Why make the idea of motivation so complicated?" My students certainly thought like that as I tried to use Atkinson's 0 to 1.0 scale to explain achievement motivation. In short, use of Atkinson's scale did not help with my advising and teaching. I needed something more straightforward and concrete, more readily connected to the process of students understanding and developing their levels of achievement motivation. I eventually decided to use a 0-100% scale instead of Atkinson's scale. Students readily took to the 0-100% measurement because it was the way that they had been evaluated since their first days in elementary school, e.g., 80% is strong, 20% is weak. The 0-100% scale was also used in many attempts to frame change in development in persons, e.g., see the initial attempts to rate personal development functioning in the Diagnostic and Statistical Manual of Mental Disorders. The 0-100% scale was only the beginning of my work to help me and students understand factors that influenced the efforts of individuals working toward success.

In studying factors that affect motivation, I came upon

two areas of research that fascinated me. Dr. John Nicholls' work was one area, wherein he theorized that persons' motivation toward an activity could be influenced by what he called "Task versus Ego Involvement." Being Task-Involved or Ego-Involved came down to how students perceived both their ability to do a task and the level of task-difficulty. A student's perceptions or "attributions" of skill level on a task could result in increased or lowered motivation. When Task-Involved, a person was motivated positively because his or her efforts were focused on step-by-step improvement toward becoming skillful or competent. Each improvement signaled getting better and, thus, increased motivation.

According to Nicholls' research, the opposite was true of achievement motivation when a person was Ego-Involved. Rather than concentrating on the task of improving, an Ego-Involved person's primary focus was on comparing their skill level to others or to perceived deficits in themselves. If skill comparison to others was one of "I am lower than . . .," an Ego-Involved person could experience lowered motivation toward a task because they saw themselves as not capable in comparison to others. Competing with others was therefore a threat, something to be avoided, and could result in "fear of failure." For Ego-Involved persons, any effort that resulted in small steps toward becoming skillful were seen as proof of being "less than" in relation to others who already were more skillful. This often leads to decreased motivation toward a task. My experience was that this was true for many ethnic minority students, like myself, who often entered university with lower skill levels in comparison to students with stronger academic backgrounds. Many years later, when studying and doing Gestalt personal development work, I heard a phrase for the first time that connected directly to Nicholls' concept of how being Ego-Involved led to lowered motivation toward a task: "Compare and despair!"

My use of the 0-100% scale to explain motivation and efforts towards success, especially for ethnic minority students, was strengthened when I connected the scale to Nicholls' concept of Task versus Ego-Involvement. Task-Involved students "got" what was meant by 100 - perfect. They "got" what was meant by 40, 50, that is, not so good. They "got" what was meant by moving from 40 to 95, hard work and step-by-step progress. Students also "got" that being Ego-Involved could result in lowered motivation because they focused too much on comparing themselves to others, rather than focusing on the task of improving their skills in a progressive manner.

Task versus Ego-Involvement

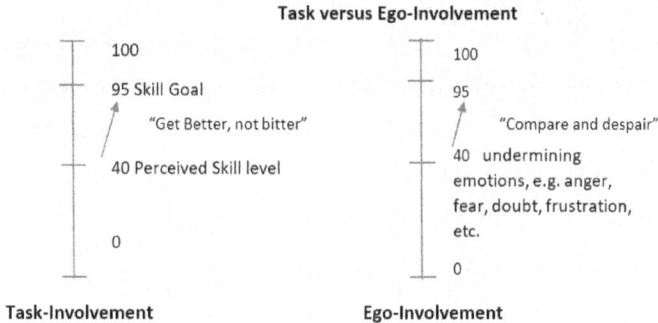

Task versus Ego Involvement- Let's say a student's skill level is low, such as 40 out of 100. If task-involved the student perceives skill level clearly and sets a goal to increase her skill level. If Ego-Involved negative comparison to others may lead to lowered motivation and effort.

Students' motivation toward a task can be lessened if a

student focuses on comparing self to others rather than focusing on the task of improving skills. In the above diagram, it can be seen that if a student rates self as low on a skill (e.g., 40), and at the same time compares him or herself to other high-skilled students or persons in their lives, negative feelings such as anger, fear, doubt, frustration, etc., often result. An added point is that at a biological level negative emotions negatively impact the brains functioning, such as focus and short-term memory. Again, negative emotions undermine achievement motivation as defined by Atkinson (1966): "All the factors that influence the direction, strength, and persistence of behavior toward a goal." Conversely, if a student is Task-Involved (the arrow is focused on the skill goal and steps required to achieve the goal), the student will be buoyed in his or her motivation by progressive improvement (every small step is a move forward!) toward the goal of developing competence (Nicholls, 1984).

Along with the ideas of John Nicholls, in my study of achievement motivation, especially the motivation of underprepared ethnic minority college students (those I saw as similar to myself when I had started college), I came upon the work of Bernard Weiner at UCLA. Weiner had developed a theory of motivation called "An Attribution Theory of Achievement and Emotion." Weiner's research showed that the "attribution" or belief a person has toward the level of difficulty of a task, and how one thinks about or perceives one's skill level toward doing a task, influence emotions which in turn affect motivation toward a task, e.g., if I think I have low skills on a task (an attribution), I can feel shame and doubt, and this will influence my motivation. Similarly, if a person sees a task as too difficult, this can influence emotions and, in turn, affect motivation toward the task, e.g., if

I think a task is too difficult, I can feel helpless or hopeless toward the task, and this will undermine my motivation toward doing and succeeding at the task.

Weiner's Attribution Theory of Achievement and Emotion

	Ability	Task-difficulty	Goal Expectancy
Perception	Low	High	Low
Feeling	Shame & doubt	Helplessness/hopelessness	*Give up (mine)*

Above are the factors identified by Weiner (1985) with respect to how an individual's attributions of ability and task-difficulty influence goal expectancies and feelings toward a particular task. For example, if a student perceives ability in writing as low, he will possibly experience negative emotions such as shame and doubt. In combination with a perception of high task difficulty regarding the task of writing and attendant negative emotions such as feeling helpless and hopeless, a student will be less motivated to attempt, persist, and complete the task of learning to write well.

I found both Atkinson's and Weiner's theories useful in my development of the 0-100% scale to help increase students' motivation and efforts towards achieving success in college. As already noted, students could rate themselves regarding how Task or Ego-Involved they were toward the tasks of academic and personal development. They could also establish standards of excellence they wanted to achieve regarding being Task-Involved. Similarly, students could rate emotional components related to being motivated, e.g., 0-100%, how much doubt do I feel? Or 0-100%, how much hopelessness do I feel? The opposite of these undermining emotions could also be rated and could be used to establish goals for improvement, including specific skills to be developed or tasks to be completed to improve motivation, e.g., 0-100%, what level of confidence (opposite of doubt) do I want to achieve and what skills do I need to develop to reach my confidence improvement goal? Or, 0-100%, what level of hope do I want to develop and what skills do I need to develop to achieve my goal of improving my level of hope? My dissertation research showed that students could indeed become more Task-Involved and improve their ability and task-difficulty attributions (self-perceptions) and that this related to improved academic performance (increased grade point average and course completion) (Rivas, 1988).

Professional Development: I develop "The 0-100% Circle of Development"

"The 0-100% Competence Method" was my initial attempt to help students organize their overall skills or personal development challenges. For example, a student could rate self with regard to skills needed to achieve his or her academic or personal development goals, both the initial level of skills as well as desired skill levels required in tasks to achieve goals (see below).

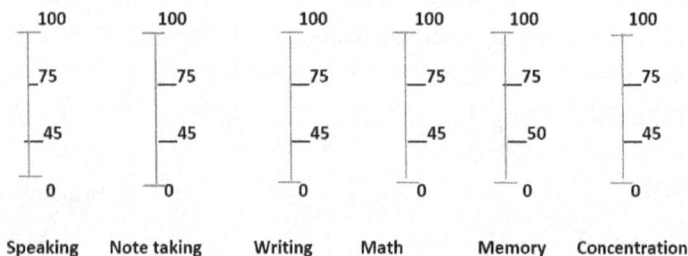

Speaking	Note taking	Writing	Math	Memory	Concentration
100	100	100	100	100	100
75	75	75	75	75	75
45	45	45	45	50	45
0	0	0	0	0	0

In 2004, I further developed the 0-100% scale by making it part of what I called the Circle of Development (unpublished manuscript, Rivas 2004). Essentially, I used a circle (recommended to me by a colleague, Pat Murray) to conceptualize how a person could view their whole self with respect to developing the skills and personality characteristics needed to become successful. The "0-100% Circle of Development" supported students to get a unified or complete picture of themselves in development and to do the following: (1) Identify personal and career goal areas considered important to complete self; (2) Establish a quantifiable achievement goal on a 0-100 scale for personality and/or career-related skill tasks; (3) Evaluate current status regarding progress toward achieving personal, academic, and career goals; (4) Assess the ongoing status of development on a particular skill, including related sub-skills, or personal characteristics necessary for achieving goals for success in life, college, and career; (5) Use the skill of self-analysis to continuously define how to change to improve skills and personal characteristics necessary to ensure achieving goals.

The 0-100% Circle of Development

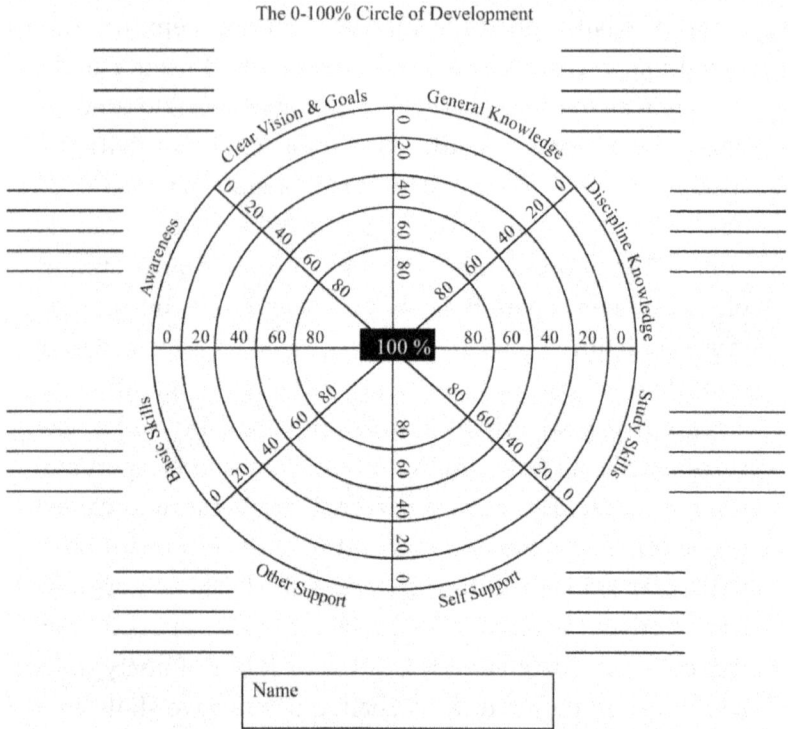

Name

The" 0-100% Circle of Development" integrates the concept of student development within college into a scheme that shows a student developing from a less to more competent position in different skill areas related to student success. In the circle, each pie slice represents a general skill area. The lines outside the circle and near each pie represent sub-skill areas, consistent with those within the 0-100% Competence Advising Model above.

An interesting use of "The 0-100% Circle of Development" is that it can depict the progress a person makes to becoming a centered and focused person. Specifically, if a person develops all her skills toward a high level, the placement of skill levels will show a "more centered person," whose skills support a strong core of being. Conversely, if the identified skills needed for a person's perceived developmental goals are varied, e.g., high, low, average, the circle will depict a person who is not centered but, instead, is "wobbly" in their current level of development.

Using "Rivas' 0-100% Circle of Development" to Organize Becoming Complete as a Person

Below I offer how to use "The 0-100% Circle of Development" to look at the task of becoming complete as a person.

Rivas' 0-100% Competence Model Applied to the Concept of Completing Self

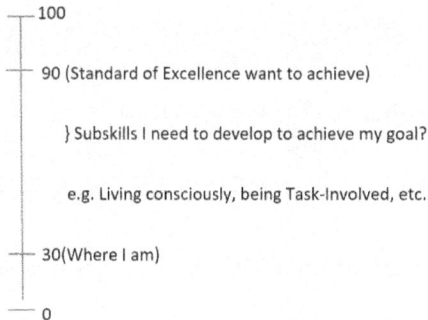

Rivas' 0-100% Competence Model Applied to the Concept of Completing Self

```
  — 100

  — 90 (Standard of Excellence want to achieve)

    } Subskills I need to develop to achieve my goal?

    e.g. Living consciously, being Task-Involved, etc.

  — 30(Where I am)

  — 0
```

How Complete Am I as a Person?

I use this model with students and community groups in personal development workshops, and I have occasionally been challenged about the use of a numerical scale as being too quantitative and not sufficiently qualitative to address the idea of human development, i.e., our life is more than numbers. My response is that I use this method because it is a scale to which students respond positively because it gives them a concrete and tangible method to organize how to assess their development in college and life, establish skills and sub-skill goals, and monitor progress toward their goals.

Truthfully, the use of the model involves approximations versus scientific specificity, but I have seen over and over that these numerical approximations are very motivating for persons to continue working toward a valued goal. In support of this, the model has been effectively used in learning centers, academic advising, and even in my Gestalt work and training in the Latino community (see SFSU Learning Center Report, 2000).

What follows is an initial depiction of what two characteristics of development in "The 0-100% Circle of Development" might look like related the task of completing self as an integrated, unified person. I have identified two areas of development that I consider important to my own search for completeness. For example, Living Consciously can be seen on the 11 o'clock outside position of the circle. Above and to the left of Living Consciously are three areas important in which to develop skills, namely, one, to be aware of what I am conscious of and how that affects my thoughts, actions, and emotions; two, learn to become aware of what I carry in my subconscious and how that influences my behavior; and, three, and much more difficult, what makes up my unconscious. I have also included being Task-Involved in life as an important aspect for achieving completeness (on the 1 o'clock outside portion of the circle). Similarly, I have

included three sub-skills related to maintaining Task-Involvement in one's life pursuits: focus on the task; avoid
comparing self to others; monitor progress toward goals.

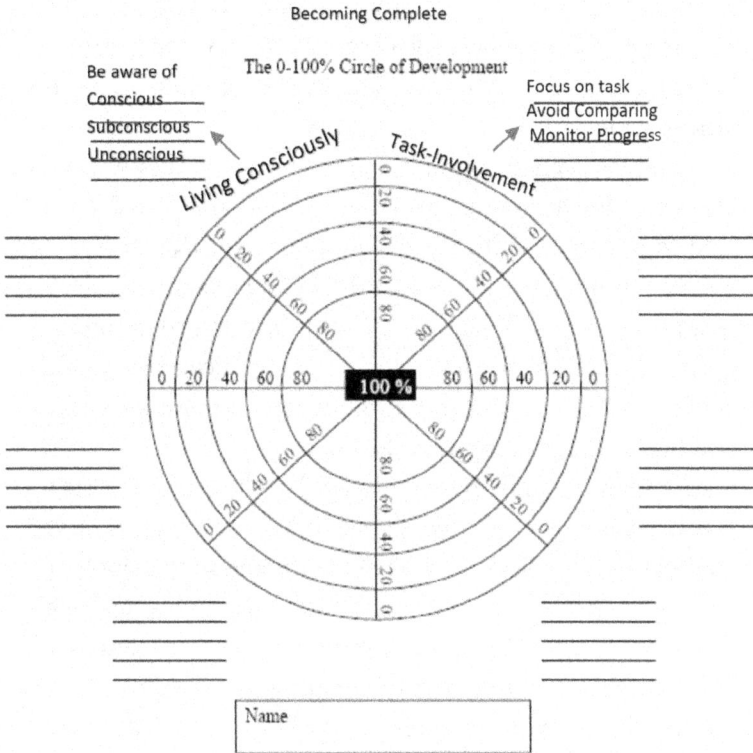

Becoming Complete

Be aware of   The 0-100% Circle of Development
Conscious   Focus on task
Subconscious   Avoid Comparing
Unconscious   Monitor Progress

Living Consciously   Task-Involvement

0 20 40 60 80   **100 %**   80 60 40 20 0

Name

I want to share what I personally consider a more com-
prehensive list of factors related to becoming complete as a
person: the first four pies in the Circle of Completeness are
from Ken Keyes' "The Twelve Pathways to Higher Consciousness:" (1) Freeing Myself (from security, sensation,
and power addictions (addictions are a shortened version
of describing strong habitual ways of thinking, feeling, and
acting — "robot-like emotional patterns") which create my

illusory version of my world; (2) Being Here Now (remembering I have everything I need to be fulfilled; assuming responsibility for the work of my development; accepting myself fully); (3) Interacting with Others (being honest in who I am so as not to hide from myself and others); (4) Discovering My Conscious Awareness (calming my rational mind; seeing all people as awakening beings; integrating my unconscious).

The fifth section contains a person's need for Skill Development (developing personal and professional skills (e.g., communication, critical thinking, etc.); (6) (Physical Self) Work at improving the peacefulness and effective functioning of my physical self; (7) Creating Brotherhood and Sisterhood (working toward equality and justice in the world); and (8) Generativity (mentoring the next generation, including one's children, grandchildren, etc.).

So, there you are, my version of how I see my efforts toward becoming a complete person. Each of the pies is rooted in the different literature I have mentioned in this book. For example, discovering my conscious awareness has to do with the work of Carl Jung, integrating the conscious with the unconscious, and with Gestalt work that builds my awareness of my unique self. With regard to Gestalt work, I see the "Gestalt Cycle of Experience" and all of the principles of Gestalt as being the energy and process necessary to develop aspects related to completing myself. Gestalt personal development work is the process of "being here-and-now," continually expanding my awareness of self, and the potentialities that I have to achieve completion as a human being.

My intent here is to provide one possible way to look at, assess, and work toward one's sense of completeness, not to argue that use of this method is how to achieve completeness. I offer you that hundreds of students and community members use this model to organize and move toward cherished goals for personal, professional, and career improvement, and even the notion of completing oneself.

I have seen over and over that use of this model increases hope in persons to continue work toward valued goals, such as achieving completeness of self in life. Again, the use of the method increases John Nicholls' "Task Involvement," where movement toward a goal, e.g., going from 40-55, increases hope and motivation toward achieving the goal. A motivational phrase in the book "Live Your Dreams" by Les Brown, a well-known African American motivational speaker, might say that movement up the 0-100% scale helps one "get better, not bitter!"

Before completing discussion of the "0-100% Circle of Development," I want to look at two concepts that relate to the use of a circle in my model. For one, the circle has been seen as a symbol that connotes wholeness or completeness. This symbol and its meaning have existed for thousands of years, and has been expressed by mandalas, which in turn can symbolize personal completeness. Second, a circle has as one of its components a center. The concept of center also has been used to describe the core of the self. In fact, Carl Jung uses the term "center" to describe a force that guides or directs the development of the Self, which he capitalizes to show that the Self is the energy that guides one's increased awareness and movement toward the unity of being.

The 0-100% Competence Model,
Gestalt Change and Growth and GEC

One my most prized personal accomplishments in applying the "0-100% Competence Advising Model" when counseling students is how I have integrated the Gestalt personal development concepts of "split" or of "me-not-me" (Schiffman,1971) and "shame binds" (Lee and Wheeler, 1996). Written at more length in the chapter entitled "Gestalt Educational Counseling" (Ali ben Yosef, 2005), I contend that very often a student's initial assessment of skill in an area related to the need for academic or personal growth in college, especially when a student is low-skilled or under-prepared for college, signals a split between what a student considers to be "of-self versus not-of-the-self" with respect to being able to learn. By way of example, many students use such phrases as "math and me don't get along," or "I don't like it" when speaking of studying science or some other subject or "Some people are good at studying foreign languages; I'm not." Specific to certain groups of students, I have found this phenomenon especially true in my extensive work with many students of color who often enter college under-prepared to meet the varied learning and personal development challenges that they will face. The "split" that I have found in students is between internalized feelings of lack of self-trust and lack of self-support to take on developmental challenges of college, which are in opposition to feelings and thoughts oriented toward attempting to succeed at such a task as improving writing, math, or science skills.

In my counseling and teaching, I have adapted the use of the "0-100% Method" to help students learn of the possible split that they experience within themselves when they try to learn and experience negative thoughts and feelings in their attempts to learn. Specifically, I discuss what I call the "Zone of Change and Growth" wherein students have to learn to support their "self" to experience and be able to handle the difficult emotions associated with changing and becoming more effective in key skill areas. For example, when a student talks about "not being able to write well" or "not being able to be confident speaking before groups," I share how the process of developing competence in any area involves learning to support oneself to handle learning or skill-building situations that are experienced as threatening. In this regard, through the use of GEC I support students to become aware of when and how in their personal development they stopped learning to support themselves to feel and express themselves with confidence. Additionally, using the 0-100% scale, the student is introduced to the notion that the identified current level of skill signals the boundary of growth for students, not the boundary of impossibility. In order to navigate this "Boundary of Change and Growth," I encourage students to learn how to support themselves rather than negate or shame themselves into not working to improve their level of efficacy in an important skill area. This learning to be supportive of self in the face of challenging learning situations is a characteristic that I reinforce in students will need to be turned to again and again as they work on developing increased competence, confidence, and "self-support" as learners.

In Diagram 4, I have drawn a graphic using the 0-100% scale that I use with students to help them become aware of the concept of "me-not-me." When I use this graphic, I talk about the safety or comfort they may feel in the "me" area of the scale, wherein they learned some level of skills related to a difficult task, e.g., basic level skills related to learning to do college-level writing. I then talk about the "Boundary of Change" and "Zone of Growth," wherein students will have to learn how to develop a high level of "self-support" in order to face difficult and challenging emotions that often accompany difficult learning challenges.

The Boundary of Change and Zone of Growth Related to the Challenge of Developing Competence as a Unique Person College-level Writing Ability

The Boundary of Change and Zone of Growth Related
to the Challenge of Developing Competence as a Unique Person

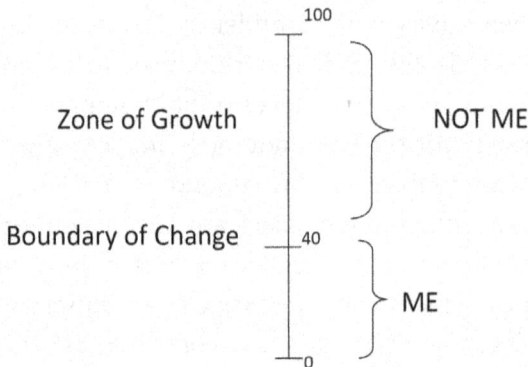

```
                         100
Zone of Growth            |        } NOT ME
Boundary of Change    __ 40
                          |        } ME
                        __ 0
```

The "Zone of Growth" is the area within the 0-100 line where a student identifies sees self as limited in ability to take on a learning task. This zone is often laden with negative emotions of fear related to doubt and often associated shame about one's ability to succeed on a task. This fear/shame and doubt often translates into lack of self-support related to either attempting or persisting on a skill task that is perceived as very difficult or overwhelming.

The task of a counselor/educator is to offer support as the student learns to develop "self-support" to persist and complete difficult learning tasks. The "Boundary of Change" signals the first step in the process of learning self-support and greater competence and confidence as a learner.

In this chapter I have shared how I have "stayed with and supported myself" to develop my professional ideals in how to support students and others to face the challenges of learning difficult developmental tasks in school and life. I am grateful to the many individuals who have supported me as I have continuously worked at developing my own "self-support" to express the uniqueness of who I am in our society. I support you to do the same!

Chapter 11

Mario's Gestalt Work to Send You on Your Way, Levitsky's Caution, and Final Words

Today I awoke thinking about this final chapter, this book, and I wondered how effective I have been in achieving my intent to write how valuable Gestalt personal development work has been for me, for others, and to share the meaning, methods, and potential of Gestalt work for you the reader. I asked myself, "0-100%, how effective have I been?" My initial response was 60. In my 0-100% scale a 60 is only a so-so rating. 'Yes, I did the task, but not so well.' I thought immediately, 'That isn't so good; what would people think about my self-rating?' What came to my mind was that I should do some Gestalt self-work to determine what my self-rating means and what the rating was communicating to me.

Is my rating a reflection of doubts and fears that I learned in my childhood, or is it a clear appraisal for how well I've achieved my original purpose? This is a very important distinction as I have pointed out in this book. Our Childhood Legacy can influence us to think, feel, and act in ways that are not consciously determined; instead, we react to life sometimes from subconscious motivations, fears, and desires developed in our early childhood, which may undermine objective thinking. So, I need to be clear from where my 0-100% rating is originating regarding how I perceive the effectiveness of this book.

To do this "Gestalt self-work" I need to see if I, as an adult, am reflecting on how well I've completed my task, or is my Childhood Legacy hurt-little-boy self the one who is coming up with my assessment? I check in my imagination to see what my little boy is doing, and instantly see an image of him reaching out for to me to pick him up. I take a deep breath. I stay with this image and what my self-rating of 60 might be saying to me. Different feelings emerge. Most figural is a tension in my forehead, then my forearms.

I close my eyes and I finish my oatmeal (sharing my here-and-now). I close my eyes to search again for my little boy. I feel strength in my upper chest and shoulders because I am feeling my truth: I need love and support. This being with my "real self" is empowering, but, still, I feel an instability in my torso and butt (recall the drawing of a child learning to stand and walk?). I choose to balance myself in my seat and I breathe more deeply, still with a mixture of instability and strength. I balance myself again, imagining different options of behavior with which to experiment. Should I work with my hurt-little-boy self or my adult self? I search again for my hurt little boy. I am instantly reminded of Robert Kegan's "The Evolving Self" book cover that depicts the development of a human being from a cellular level to a fully developed adult. What I see is an image of a child over time becoming an adult.

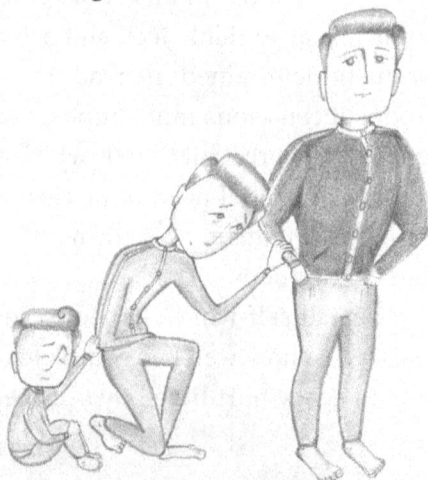

My "here-and-now experience" is that I am evolving in the clarity and completeness of my being. I get up to get my iPhone to take a picture of Kegan's book cover. I feel a mixture of balance, strength, and nervous weakness in my legs. I go and take a bite of my chicken sausage and have a sip of coffee. My chest is expanded and my shoulders are square as I walk to my bedroom. I am in the present. I close my eyes to see my little boy and I breathe more deeply, even though now in my imagination I do not see my little boy nor the Kegan graphic. I only feel myself, here and now, within the small cottage-like house in which I live.

My attention moves to my garden outside my window. I feel a slight dizziness in my forehead. I tell myself, "Speak from that dizziness, Mario." (This is an example self-therapy as taught by Muriel Schiffman in her book "Gestalt Self-Therapy.") I move my neck to feel my life. I breathe more deeply. "I am here in the present! I am being the self I want to be here and now and at a self-rating of 95. I am all my reactions . . . *Saber, Entender, Sentir, Escoger y Hacer.* I am being the Gestalt Cycle of Experience . . . sensing, being aware, mobilizing my energy, acting, having contact with the reality of my being. In response to these thoughts, what becomes figural for me is a strength in my legs. I breathe more deeply. I want to walk, be with my recently planted tomato seeds. I do so, and see that my seedling tomatoes are "working" to become young plants.

Walking back to my computer, I want to experiment with my "Warrior-self," a piece of Gestalt personal development work that Dr. Lou Grey from the Bay Area Gestalt Institute once did with me. I remember her saying to me as I began to tear in her Gestalt workshop, "I know you can access your crying, hurt child self. Let's now get in contact with the warrior in you." I slip out of my flip-flops and assume the warrior pose. I feel the strength of the grass, the earth beneath my feet. I bend my knees, move about as if an ancient warrior. I am here, experimenting, and being, and sharing the goodness and strength of life around me and within me. I look for my little boy and I see him with his hands on his hips like me — balanced in his being. I also see Kegan's graphic of the evolving self. I breathe deeply and I feel an integrity, a unity of self, a completeness of being.

I am back from my little bit of personal work. I stayed with my experience. I am more complete in my being, knowing more of the reality of life in me and around me. With respect to the Gestalt Cycle of Experience, I came in "contact" with myself in each moment, and did not shy away from the experience of my self. Again, I ask myself, "0-100%, how well have I accomplished my goal in writing this book?" My answer: "I have done what I have done; I have been faithful to my intention, and I have made a very good effort." How does this translate to a 0-100% rating? For me, an 80, pretty good, but not totally great. Still, I think and feel I did a more than worthwhile, creditable job.

Wow! I feel I should go back and rewrite my book from the beginning in this voice. But, no, because that would not show the progression or development of my communicating with you. I'll see about writing this way in the future... What follows is what I wrote before this morning as a book ending. I keep it and share it because then you can see how my attempt to communicate with you can vary. Our actions vary because as persons we are varied as we go through our lives, working every day to get to know our true self— to become complete.

I was born as a unified organism and I have been

bequeathed from millions of years of evolution with the physical resources necessary to experience the realities of the social and physical world and to learn to live effectively with clarity and satisfaction. Still, in childhood I had to go through a vulnerable period when my organism, my "self," had to be supported from the outside, "other support," to develop inner support, "self-support," so as to experience my natural being as part of the world and universe, within and around me. This is when my challenge to achieve completeness began, my birthright to experience life, again, with effectiveness, clarity, and satisfaction.

At the beginning of this book, I shared how my negative childhood experiences, especially with my abusive father, created within my biopsychological self (mind and body), a theme. This theme influenced and to a great extent directed how I thought, felt, and acted in the world, too often with doubt, shame, panic, and lack of self-worth. I called this "My Childhood Legacy." My Childhood Legacy then combined with my Latino experience in the U.S.A., where I also experienced an instability because my experience was that I was not an acceptable part of our society. I shared how this Childhood Legacy projected itself into my adult personality and diverted my "self" from my "birthright to achieve completeness." Rather than having developed as a unified and complete organism, I was an organism, a la Perls, filled with holes, splits, lack of harmonious coordination, and negative internalized feelings. I had developed these blocks to my natural completeness through negative learning. Through positive re-learning, though, I would regain my human birthright to be complete.

Primarily through my Gestalt personal development work I progressively freed myself and began my journey to greater personal awareness. To me, this journey is akin to what Robert Kegan calls the "activity that a human being is." Here we arrive at the crux of what for me is the meaning of achieving completeness. Our unique human activity is our sentience, our ability to experience the world with our senses and to construct our individual meaning of life. This "meaning-making" can be termed as either "real" or "not real." "Real" means that we honestly experience our meaning-making in life as truth for us, a truth that supports us to experience life with increasing clarity and effectiveness.

"Not real" is when we turn away from seeing the truth of our lives; this is when we do not provide self-support to be and express ourselves with truth and honesty. Andre Gide, a well-known French philosopher, said, "The belief that is truth for me . . . is that which allows me the best use of my strength, the best means of putting my virtues into practice." Here, the word virtues point to personal strengths to act out our true self. I call this our "Hand-on-Heart" experience. In short, I have seen over and over that when I or others invoke true personal values and beliefs, we inevitably place our hand on our chest and over our hearts. It's as if when we are being truthful to our real self we have a feeling in our heart of strength, inspiration, and clarity of experience.

This "Hand-on-Heart" phenomenon is important to achieving completeness as a unique human being. Our uniqueness is our true self, our real self, our "Hand-on-Heart" self. This requires that we clear away all social conditioning of what we should be or how we should live life. We must liberate ourselves from our past external conditioning, especially our Childhood Legacy, so that we may complete a self that experiences and acts on life with more and more clarity based on our uniqueness.

Dr. Miles Neale, a Buddhist therapist practicing in New York, in his YouTube presentation titled "Spiritual Awakening for a Brighter Future," uses a simple analogy to explain how our learned conditioning influences our perceptions of life. He describes how the mirrors in a funhouse can make it seem that we are other than we are: fatter, skinnier, taller. We know, of course, that these images are not real. However, in life we often learn through social conditioning, especially during the vulnerable time of childhood, to perceive life and ourselves inaccurately, e.g., we may perceive ourselves as not good enough or lacking in some way in comparison to others. Unlike the experience with the funhouse mirrors, we do not readily see that our conditioned negative perceptions of self and life are too often illusions that get in the way of having clear perceptions toward our life experiences. It is these inaccurate perceptions that we must shatter to liberate ourselves so as to look with clarity as to who we are, and, most importantly, how we want to author our real self.

Dr. Abe Levitsky used to chide me, "Gestalt personal development work isn't everything!" No, Abe, but to me Gestalt work, and in my case, the use of Gestalt Educational Counseling, is crucial for liberating ourselves from inaccurate perceptions and beliefs that come from our Childhood Legacies. By being aware and making use of the Gestalt Cycle of Experience, we can learn that if in every moment we make it a habit to support ourselves with the "Hand-on Heart" truth of what we experience with our senses and mind, we can think, feel, and act more clearly our unique selves. Achieving completeness is our ability to develop a level of awareness in life, what Gestaltists call "creative indifference," wherein we are supportive and receptive and not biased for how we truly think, feel, and want to act in life.

Also, in deference to Dr. Levitsky, I acknowledge the power of what Carl Jung has bequeathed us regarding what it means to achieve completeness as a person: to develop a whole, complete Self, we need to integrate our conscious self with our subconscious and unconscious self. We must integrate into our complete Self what we perceive as reality with our senses with that part of our Self, our subconscious, wherein we learned to block our ability to see, understand, and react to experiences that threaten our sense of self, e.g., my cartoon image of chaos, and with our unconscious, which is our evolutionary inheritance of our developing from animal to human.

Different from my Gestalt personal work this clarifying of my conscious self with my subconscious and unconscious self is a task I have recently begun working to understand more clearly. Jung wrote that our unconscious can only be accessed indirectly and can only be inferred because the unconscious can never be truly known. Still, we can get a good idea of our unconscious, especially what Jung termed the personal subconscious, which is that part of our unconscious that we develop because of our unique childhood experiences. This is part of what I have called our Childhood Legacy.

Staying with the importance of understanding our subconscious in order to achieve completeness, I turn to a book by Timothy Wilson. In "Strangers to Ourselves," Wilson shares a great amount of recent social-psychological research documenting how we do indeed have a subconscious self, and that our subconscious self directs our actions very often in ways not known to us. Dr. Wilson calls this the "adaptive unconscious," which is related to Hanson and Mendius' hidden memories from our childhood experiences. In the end, much like Carl Jung, Wilson notes that by honest self-observation we can know aspects of our subconscious, but that we cannot fully know our unconscious. I need to learn more in this area.

Again, in closing, I come back to the importance of Gestalt personal development work as being a powerful and useful process to support us to move toward knowing and being our true self. This process, indeed, is what I have arrived at as what it means to achieve completeness as a person. Life presents us with so many options or possibilities for how to be. However, the options are only secondary to what it means to be complete as a human being. Our most complete self is a self which is aware of our ability to feel, think, and act in unique ways, in ways that may change as we live life, but in ways where we develop the awareness to not lose our ability to know that we are an integral part of the vast universe that surrounds us!

Bibliography

Adler, Mortimer and Charles Van Doren. "How to Read a Book." Simon & Shuster, New York, NY. 1972.

Baca, Jimmy Santiago. "A Place to Stand." Grove Press, New York. NY. 2001.

Berne, Eric. "Transactional Analysis in Psychotherapy." Ballantine Books, New York. 1961.

Berne, Eric. "Games People Play – The Psychology of Human Relationships." Grove Press, Inc., New York, NY. 1964.

Branden, Nathaniel. "The Psychology of Self Esteem." Jossey Bass, San Francisco, Ca. 1969.

Branden, Nathaniel. "The Six Pillars of Self Esteem." Bantam Books, New York, NY. 1994.

Brown, T., & Rivas, M. "The Prescriptive Relationship in Academic Advising as an Appropriate Developmental Intervention with Multicultural Populations. NACADA Journal, 1994.

Erikson, Erik. "Childhood and Society." W.W. Norton, New York, NY. 1950.

Erikson, Erik. And Erikson, Joan. "The Life Cycle Completed." W.W. Norton and Company, New York, New York.1997

Evan, Richard. "Dialogue with Erik Erikson." Harper and Row. New York, NY. 1967.

Fromm, Erich. "The Art of Loving." Harper & Row, New York, NY. 1956.

Goldstein, Kurt. "The Organism-A Holistic Approach to Biology Derived from Pathological Data in Man." Zone Books, New York, 2000.

Gonzales, Rodolfo. Ýo Soy Juaquin." Bantam Books, New York. 1972.

Hanson, Rick and Mendius, Richard. "Buddhas's Brain – The Practical Neuroscience of Happiness, Love and Wisdom" New Harbinger Publications, Inc. Oakland, California, 2009.

Harris, Thomas. "I'm Ok – You're Ok." Avon Books, New York. 1973.

Heller, Joseph. "Bodywise." Wingbow Press, Berkeley, Ca. 1991.

Horney, Karen. "Our Inner Conflicts." W.W. Norton & Company, Inc. New York, NY. 1945.

Jourard, Sidney. "The Transparent Self." Princeton, N.J.; Nostrum, Co. Inc., 1964.

Kegan, Robert. "The Evolving Self." Harvard University Press, Boston, Mass. 1982.

Kegan, Robert and Lahey, Lisa. Immunity to Change. Harvard Business School Publishing Corporation, Boston, Mass. 2009.

Keleman, Stanley. "Your Body Speaks Its Mind." Center Press, Berkeley, Ca. 1981.

Keyes, Ken, Jr. "Handbook to Higher Consciousness." Living Love Publications, Coos Bay, Or., 1975.

Kopp, Sheldon. "If You Meet the Buddha on the Road, Kill Him – The Pilgrimage of Psychotherapy Patients." Bantam, Books, New York, NY. 1976.

Lee, Robert. "Shame and the Gestalt Model." "In the Voice of Shame- Silence and Connection in Psychotherapy." Edited by Lee, Robert, Wheeler, Gordon. Gestalt Press, The Analytic Press, New Jersey. 2003

Levine, E.S., & Padilla, A.M. "Crossing Cultures in Therapy: Pluralistic Counseling for the Hispanic." Monterey, CA: Brooks/Cole Publishing Co., 1980.

Maslow, Abraham. "Toward a Psychology of Being." Van Nostrum Reinhold Company, New York, New York. 1968.

Neale, Miles. "Spiritual Awakening for a Brighter Future." Watkinsbooks.com. 2010

Nicholls, John. G. "Achievement Motivation: Conceptions of personality, subjective experience, task choice, and performance." "Psychological Review," 91, 328-349.

Peck, Scott. "The Road Less Traveled." Simon and Schuster, New York, NY. 1978.

Perls, Fritz. "Gestalt Therapy Verbatim." Real People Press, Lafayette, CA.: Real People Press, 1969.

Perls, Fritz. "In and Out of the Garbage Pail." Real People Press, Lafayette, CA.: Real People Press, 1969.

Perls, Frederick. "Theory and Technique of Personality Integration." In "Gestalt Is." Edited by John O. Stevens. Real People Press, Maob, Utah. 1975.

Plotnik, Rod and Kouyoumdjiam, Haig. "Introduction to Psychology." Wadsworth Cengage Learning. Belmont, CA. 2011.

Polster, Irving and Miriam. "Gestalt Therapy Integrated." Bruner/Mazel Publishers. New York, New York. 1973.

Powell, John. "Why Am I Afraid to Tell You Who I Am?" Argus Communications, London.1969.

Reich, Wilhelm. "Character Analysis." Ferrar Strauss and Giroux, New York, NY. 1933.

Rendon, Laura. "Validating Culturally Diverse Students: Toward a New Model of Learning and Student Development." Innovative Higher Education. Vol. 19, No. 1, fall, 1994.

Rivas, A. Mario. "Gestalt Educational Counseling." In "The Bridge-Dialogue Across Cultures," Talia Levine Bar Joseph, Editor. Gestalt Institute Press, Metairie, New Orleans, La., 2005.

Rivas, A. Mario. "An Exploratory Study of a Group Intervention for Underprepared Minority University Students." Minneapolis, Minnesota: Doctoral Thesis, 1988.

Rogers, Carl. "Freedom to Learn," Charles E. Merrill, Publishing, Co. Columbus, Ohio, 1969.

Rogers, Carl. "Person to Person." Houghton Mifflin, Co., Boston, Mass. 1961.

Schofield, William. "Psychotherapy: The Purchase of Friendship." Routledge, . 1986.

Schutz, William. "The Human Element." Jossey-Bass, San Francisco, Ca. 1994.

Schutz, William. "Joy – Expanding Human Awareness." Grove Press, Inc. New York, NY. 1967.

Schiffman, Muriel. "Gestalt Self Therapy." Wingbow Press. Berkeley, Ca. 1971.

Steele, Claude. "Whistling Vivaldi: How Stereotypes Affect Us and What We Can Do" W.W. Norton and Company. New York, New York. 2011.

Teachworth, Anne. "Why We Pick the Mates We Do." The Gestalt Institute Press, Metairie, La. 2003.

Van Der Kolk. "The Body Keeps the Score – Brain, Mind and Body in the Healing of Trauma.

Penguin Books, New York, New York. 2014

Weiner, Bernard. "Attributional Theory of Achievement and Emotion." Psychological Review (92, 548-573), 1985.

Wheeler, Gordon. "Gestalt Reconsidered." Gardner Press, Inc., New York, NY. 1991.

Zinker, Joseph. "Creative Process in Gestalt Therapy." New York: Vintage Books, 1977.

About the Author

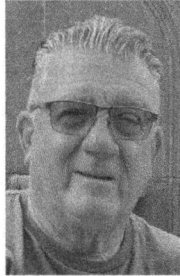

Mario Rivas, Ph.D., is a first-generation Latino in the USA who overcame personal and societal struggles to attain personal and career fulfillment that honors his uniqueness as an integral member of our society. Raised on welfare by a single Spanish-speaking mother who was a maid, Dr. Rivas used his mother's and brother's love and caring to help him overcome initial failure in community college to eventually earn a Bachelor's Degree in Psychology at California State University, Hayward, a Master's Degree in Counseling from San Francisco State University, and a Ph.D. in Counseling and Student Personnel Psychology from the University of Minnesota, Minneapolis. Dr. Rivas presents a self who because of his diverse ethnic and social experiences cares for and works for a society that supports all peoples to find goodness and truth in themselves and others.

Dr. Rivas is an accomplished speaker who has given hundreds of presentations across the USA and Puerto Rico, specifically of the following type: conference key note addresses, College Graduation speeches, seminars, organizational trainings and teaching regarding theories and methods for advising college students to achieve success in their studies and of Gestalt Personal Development approaches to empower individuals' unique personal development. Dr. Rivas has taught Psychology and Counseling at the undergraduate levels in Community College and Universities and graduate counseling at the University level. Before retiring as a tenured professor in Psychology from Merritt College in Oakland, California, where he also served as Academic Senate President for 4 years, Dr. Rivas held extended posts as Vice President of Student Services at Berkeley City College and Associate Dean of Undergraduate Studies at San Francisco State University. Dr. Rivas has and continues to do community work in Spanish and English in the San Francisco-Oakland Bay Area, sharing his knowledge of Gestalt psychology and personal development and continues to mentor students of color who wish to pursue careers in Psychology.

ABOOKS

ALIVE Book Publishing and ALIVE Publishing Group
are imprints of Advanced Publishing LLC,
3200 A Danville Blvd., Suite 204, Alamo, California 94507

Telephone: 925.837.7303
alivebookpublishing.com